SANDTRAY
THERAPY

Sandtray Therapy is an essential book for professionals and students interested in incorporating this unique modality into work with clients of all ages. The third edition includes information on integrating neurological aspects of trauma and sandtray, updates per the DSM-5, and a new chapter on normative studies of the use of sandtray across the lifespan. As in previous editions, readers will find that the book is replete with handouts, images, examples, and resources for use in and out of the classroom. The authors' six-step protocol guides beginners through a typical session, including room setup, creation and processing of the sandtray, cleanup, post-session documentation, and much more.

Linda E. Homeyer, PhD, LPC-S, RPT-S, is a professor of professional counseling at Texas State University and director of the Door of Hope Counseling Center in New Braunfels, Texas.

Daniel S. Sweeney, PhD, LMFT, LPC, RPT-S, is a professor of counseling, director of the clinical mental health counseling program, and director of the NW Center for Play Therapy Studies at George Fox University in Portland, Oregon.

SANDTRAY THERAPY

A Practical Manual

Third Edition

Linda E. Homeyer
Daniel S. Sweeney

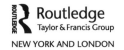
Routledge
Taylor & Francis Group

NEW YORK AND LONDON

Third edition published 2017
by Routledge
711 Third Avenue, New York, NY 10017

and by Routledge
2 Park Square, Milton Park, Abingdon, Oxon, OX14 4RN

Routledge is an imprint of the Taylor & Francis Group, an informa business

First edition published by Lindan Press 1998
Second edition published by Routledge 2010

Library of Congress Cataloging-in-Publication Data
Names: Homeyer, Linda, author. | Sweeney, Daniel S., author.
Title: Sandtray therapy : a practical manual / Linda E. Homeyer, Daniel S. Sweeney.
Description: Third edition. | New York, NY : Routledge, 2016. | Includes bibliographical references and index.
Identifiers: LCCN 2016004261 | ISBN 9781138950054 (hbk : alk. paper) | ISBN 9781138950047 (pbk : alk. paper) | ISBN 9781315651903 (ebk)
Subjects: LCSH: Play therapy. | Sandplay—Therapeutic use. | Sand tables.
Classification: LCC RJ505.P6 H66 2016 | DDC 618.92/891653—dc23
LC record available at http://lccn.loc.gov/2016004261

ISBN: 978-1-138-95005-4 (hbk)
ISBN: 978-1-138-95004-7 (pbk)
ISBN: 978-1-315-65190-3 (ebk)

Typeset in Times LT Std
by Apex CoVantage, LLC

Contents

About the Authors

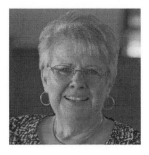

Linda E. Homeyer, Ph.D., LPC-S, RPT-S, is a professor in the Professional Counseling Program of the Department of Counseling, Leadership, Adult Education and School Psychology at Texas State University in San Marcos, Texas. Linda is a Texas Licensed Professional Counselor and Supervisor and Registered Play Therapist and Supervisor. She developed the play therapy training program at Texas State including the first play therapy course available by distance learning. Linda is a frequent presenter at professional conferences and training throughout the United States and internationally. As an advocate for children and play therapy, she helped organize the first state branch of the Association for Play Therapy (APT) and served on the Texas Association for Play Therapy board of directors in various positions. Linda also served on the Association for Play Therapy (APT) board of directors for six years. Linda received APT's *Lifetime Achievement Award* (2013) and was designated a *Director Emerita* (2014). Linda coauthored *Play Therapy in Malaysia* (2015), *Play Therapy Intervention with Children's Problems* (2005) and *The World of Play Therapy Literature* (2003), as well as numerous chapters and journal articles. She coedited the book *The Handbook of Group Play Therapy* (1999) with Daniel Sweeney. Her books have been translated into Russian, Korean, Chinese, and Spanish. Linda continues to teach and write in the areas of play therapy, sandtray therapy, and children who have been sexually abused. Her latest area of interest is spirituality and religion in play therapy and sandtray therapy. Linda also serves children and families as Director of the Door of Hope Counseling Center in New Braunfels, Texas, which she established in 2013.

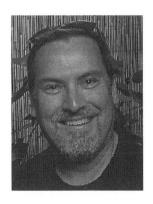

Daniel S. Sweeney, Ph.D., LMFT, LPC, ACS, RPT-S, is a Professor of Counseling, Director of the Clinical Mental Health Counseling program, and Director of the Northwest Center for Play Therapy Studies at George Fox University in Portland, Oregon. He is a past board member and president of the Association for Play Therapy, and currently serves on the editorial board for the *International Journal of Play Therapy*. As a licensed marital and family therapist, licensed professional counselor, and registered play therapist-supervisor, Daniel maintains a small private practice and has extensive clinical and supervision experience in working with children, couples, and families in a variety of settings. He has presented at numerous national and international conferences—on six continents—on the topics of sandtray therapy, play therapy, filial therapy, and trauma interventions. Daniel has multiple publications, and is author or co-author of several books, including *Play Therapy Interventions with Children's Problems* (2005), *Counseling Children Through the World of Play* (1997), *The Handbook of Group Play Therapy* (1999), and *Group Play Therapy: A Dynamic Approach* (2014). His books have been translated into Chinese, Korean, and Russian. Daniel and his wife live in Portland, Oregon near their four adult children and grandchildren.

Foreword

I have been incorporating sandtray or sandplay therapy into my work with children and families since the late 1970's, and I continue to be amazed at the scope and breadth of its reach. I continue introducing both new students and seasoned therapists to this amazing psychotherapeutic tool, and welcome them to take the personal journey of building their own sand tray so they might understand first-hand the amazing power of sand therapy. Time and again, I join the wonder and joy of students and professionals as they become enthralled with this process. The most consistent outcome of professional training is how actively mental health professionals from diverse theoretical backgrounds become enthusiasts of sandtray therapy, quickly collecting miniatures, building or purchasing sand trays, sharing sandtray stories, and creating an environment in which their sand therapy work can evolve. Sandtray therapy is a fluid and evocative nonverbal therapy process that can both enlighten and confront the sandtray creator. Thus, it has amazing potential to override resistance and provoke the unconscious to become available for externalizing and then processing even the most difficult or challenging experiences. When metaphorical and symbolic elements emerge in the sand tray, therapeutic work becomes more accessible and possible and transformative experiences can occur.

Thousands of professionals across the country have become more and more aware of the potential benefits of sandtray therapy. Two major theories influence the type of sandtray therapy that is used: Jungian (*sandplay*) and Freudian (*sandtray*). Dora Kalff, a Jungian analyst, was responsible for most of the early exposure of sandplay in the United States. She was an inspiring and dedicated analyst who coined the phrase "free and protected space," a concept that is very central in sandplay therapists.

Margaret Lowenfeld was a pediatrician, influenced by Freudian principles, who first designed a 'magic box' with children's miniature toys for free play, and later included shelves with both sand and water in her office. Children transferred the miniature toys to the sand boxes and thus, created sandtray therapy, a story that fills my heart with joy. Although these two women were friends and communicated with each other about their respective sand work over the years, sandtray therapy is characterized by the therapist's more directive approach and use of interpretation and guidance. A contemporary understanding is that sandtray therapy is used with couples, families, groups, and that mental health professionals who use sandtray therapy come from many diverse theoretical orientations and incorporated more directive approaches, including active interpretation.

Linda and Daniel take an integrated approach to sandtray therapy, viewing the process as cross-theoretical and incorporating a wide array of techniques. Having said this, they have a deep respect for basic sandplay tenets. Recognizing the crucial need to establish a safe container—that 'free and protected space'—both in the therapy room and in the sand tray, they embrace what Jung shared: "Often the hands know how to solve a riddle with which the intellect has wrestled in vain." While often taking Lowenfeld's approach to creating 'worlds' in the sand tray, Linda and Daniel also see great value in sandplay's focus on the importance of symbols. They acknowledge that these symbols can indeed be a bridge between the client's inner and outer worlds. In taking this more inclusive view, they also build some professional bridges between all professionals who value and incorporate the use of sand therapy in their practices.

In the United States, there is more training and literature regarding sandplay therapy; however, many mental health professionals and educators are attracted to a less structured use of sandtray therapy with a variety of populations and in a variety of settings. Thus, sandtray therapy holds more promise across settings and theoretical orientations.

Many mental health professionals and educators feel great excitement when exposed to sandtray therapy, yet they are often unable to find adequate training resources—thus, they simply begin to do the work without suitable preparation. This book is a fantastic first step for those unfamiliar with sandtray therapy, if it is studied with serious attention. It offers a solid foundation upon which to build. The writers are clear on this point: Their work is part of the preparation, but not a replacement for more in-depth training, and especially, having personal experiences with sand therapy and obtaining good supervision (accountability).

I have always been a loyal fan of Homeyer and Sweeney's book, *Sandtray Therapy: A Practical Manual* since its initial publication in 1998. I opened this third edition with great anticipation and hoped that it would be more than a minor revision. I was so pleased to find a page-turner, packed with information that is practical, accessible, and immediately useful. This book continues to be the single text I recommended to anyone wanting an introduction to sandtray therapy, and I am once again filled with excitement to see this manual go into a third edition.

The chapters continue to be inviting, filled with sound advice, and informative. The new chapter on developmental issues and assessment across the lifespan is a very helpful addition. The chapters about group work and couple and family work have not just been revised but include new interventions that are innovative and stimulating. I have done lots of family and group work and there are some great novel ideas for engaging children and adults. I truly enjoyed reading this book and felt motivated to try some of the activities that are shared. The chapter on trauma is not only updated, but also demonstrates the authors' facility with complex issues of neuroscience and the effects of trauma on the brain. There is a brilliant explanation of how and why sand therapy can assist in reversing the impact of trauma. Additionally, with the continued emphasis on evidence-based practices, I was actually heartened to see that more sandtray therapists have ventured into the world of research and that the results are promising.

This book is an awesome contribution to a basic understanding of the potential of sand therapy and provides an ethical and careful consideration of many aspects of providing sandtray therapy. This third edition has included the many current changes in the mental health field in general, like the incorporation of neuroscience and the importance of attachment work in any therapy work done with children.

Having done a great deal of training myself, I recognize that many mental health professionals and educators highly value verbal communication. Although the authors point out the many ways that sandtray therapy can serve as an alternative method of communication (primarily nonverbal), it can also be a conduit for reflection and verbal dialogue by client and therapist, particularly after a strong therapy relationship has been established. The authors provide many ways for therapists to interact verbally with the tray, encouraging them to stay in the metaphor and not make too many direct interpretations. Thus, this book has something for everyone and definitely achieves its' goal of introducing readers to myriad practical applications of sandtray therapy. I highly recommend it and as mentioned earlier, it has been my first recommendation to anyone considering sand therapy work in general, and sandtray work specifically.

I encourage the reader to purchase and review this lovely and useful text. I love it for its accessible language, responsible reviews of the literature, creativity, and obvious passion for the work. Thank you Linda and Daniel for this great contribution to our knowledge and clear directives for application!

Eliana Gil, Founder and Senior Clinical Consultant
Gil Institute for Trauma Recovery and Education
Fairfax, VA

1

Introduction

An abused child comes in for therapy, terrified and hiding behind the legs of her foster parent. She has been sexually victimized and won't talk. An angry adolescent is compelled to come in for counseling because of his delinquent behavior. He sees himself as a mandated client and refuses to talk. A couple on the brink of separation seeks counseling as a last result. They won't or can't communicate with each other, much less a therapist. A family walks into your office in crisis, with noncompliant and acting out children, and parents who feel helpless and hopeless. The family system is crumbling. What do you do?

Our training and experience is similar to many of the readers of this book. Many therapists would suggest (insist?) in these situations that the clients must *talk* about what has happened to them, as well as what they are currently experiencing. What is the classic counseling question?—"How does that make you feel?" Of course, these clients must verbalize their pain and frustration in order to process issues and begin healing. Really?

Is it possible that clients might not be able to verbally express their stories and the accompanying pain through verbalization alone? Our experience, and the literature on sandtray therapy (see Chapter 12) and play therapy (Bratton, 2015; Ray, 2015), however, considers moving beyond this narrow position. We would suggest that for therapists working with clients who have experienced chaos, turmoil, and trauma—a nonverbally based psychotherapeutic intervention is not just helpful, but necessary: An intervention that has expressive and projective qualities. Our favorite: Sandtray therapy.

Sandtray therapy is an expressive and projective therapy that has the unique and extraordinary quality of being considerably flexible and adaptive. It can integrate a wide variety of theoretical and technical psychotherapeutic approaches. It can be nondirective or directive, completely nonverbal or verbally assisted, and incorporate techniques from a wide spectrum of counseling approaches. This makes sandtray therapy a truly cross-theoretical intervention.

It should be emphasized that we believe sandtray is cross-theoretical, not atheoretical. Sandtray therapy theory and techniques should always be theoretically based. Sweeney (2011) asserted that theory is always important, but theory without technique is basically philosophy. At the same time techniques may be quite valuable, but techniques without theory are reckless, and could be damaging. Sweeney (2011) further asserted:

> All therapists are encouraged to ponder some questions regarding employing techniques: (a) Is the technique developmentally appropriate? [which presupposes that developmental capabilities are a key therapeutic consideration]; (b) What theory underlies the technique? [which presupposes that techniques should be theory-based]; and (c) What is the therapeutic intent in employing a given technique? [which presupposes that having specific therapeutic intent is clinically and ethically important]. (p. 236)

Both theories and techniques will be discussed in following chapters.

DEVELOPMENTAL CONSIDERATIONS

Sandtray therapy is used with clients across the developmental lifespan. When working with children, either individually or in a family system, we must recognize that they do not communicate in the same way that adults do. Children do not have the cognitive or verbal maturity to communicate in counseling in the manner as adults' converse. Children communicate through play. Landreth (2012) suggested: "Children's play can be more fully appreciated when recognized as their natural medium of communication . . . for children to 'play out' their experiences and feelings is the most natural dynamic and self-healing process in which children can engage" (p. 9).

Developmental psychology supports the use of play rather than talk as a means for communicating with children. Play, like children, is preoperational. Since children do not possess the developmental or intellectual sophistication to participate in adult, verbally based therapies, it should be concluded that the very nature of childhood is incompatible with the formal operations of adult counseling. To require a child to participate in traditional adult therapy sends a very clear message: "We are the experts. We expect you to come up to our level of communication. We are unwilling to enter your world."

We have both heard an international expert on child sexual abuse present at conferences. In one presentation, this expert stated that the first thing that he requires sexually abused children to do in therapy is to draw a picture of the perpetrator. Beside the incredibly intrusive and potentially re-traumatizing nature of this intervention—is anyone caught by of the use of the word "requires"? Haven't sexual abuse survivors already been *required* to do more than enough in the context of the victimization experience? Sandtray therapists should never be this dishonoring and demanding.

We also believe that these fundamental truths apply to adolescents and adults who have experienced conflict or trauma. In many ways, trauma—which must be generally defined, since the severity of trauma covers a broad spectrum, and the response of various clients covers an equally broad spectrum—is preoperational. It impacts people of any age at a very basic and sensory level, which does not lend itself to sophistication, categorization, or reason. Akin to requiring a drawing of the perpetrator, to *require* a person of any age to verbalize when in an emotional crisis is not just unfair, it may in fact be re-traumatizing. One way in which this has been illustrated when conducting training on play and sandtray therapy has been to ask the audience for a volunteer to stand up and share his or her most embarrassing and traumatizing sexual experience. After the nervous laughter has subsided, the point is made: "Isn't this what we do with clients who have been molested whom we ask, 'Tell us what happened to you?'" (Sweeney, 1997).

A TRAUMA INTERVENTION

The neurobiological effects of trauma will be more fully discussed in Chapter 10, but a few summary comments are important here. The effects of trauma are most pronounced on the midbrain, where the limbic system resides—the primary seat of emotions. The executive functioning of the brain, primarily located in the frontal cortex, often experiences a level of deactivation for trauma victims. This also occurs for the Broca's area of the brain, which is responsible for speech. So, when people recall their trauma (which is an expectation for many therapeutic approaches), there is a decreased ability to cognitively process material, a decreased ability to even verbalize, and an increased level of emotional material. Expecting clients to talk at this point may be substantially difficult, if not impossible. An expressive intervention like sandtray therapy is arguably a wonderful fit.

Also, the very fundamental and sensory aspects to trauma indicate the need for a sensory-based treatment such as sandtray therapy. Perhaps the reader has noticed that the diagnostic criteria for posttraumatic stress disorder in the DSM-5 (American Psychiatric Association, 2013) is largely sensory based—note the diagnostic criteria of re-experiencing, avoidance, negative cognitions and mood, and arousal. There is a fundamental recognition that trauma in and of itself is sensory based. In fact, many researchers note that traumatic memories are encoded not only in the brain, but within the body as well (Malchiodi, 2015; van der Kolk, 2014). It would seem to make sense, therefore, that the treatment for traumatized children, adolescents, and adults should also be sensory based. "Talk" therapy approaches do not meet this criteria; sandtray therapy does.

This sensory base builds the relational foundation of sandtray therapy as well. When the therapist and client(s) are not limited by verbalization, the therapeutic alignment necessary to approach and process traumatic material is enhanced. The importance of relationship is also fundamental to neurologically processing trauma. Perry and Pate (1994) emphasize this point:

> It is the 'relationship' which enables access to parts of the brain involved in social affiliation, attachment, arousal, affect, anxiety regulation and physiological hyper-reactivity (Perry & Pate, 1994, p. 142). Therefore, the elements of therapy which induce positive changes will be the relationship and the ability of the child to re-experience traumatic events in the context of a safe and supportive relationship.

SANDTRAY THERAPY, PLAY, AND THERAPEUTIC RELATIONSHIP

This focus on relationship cannot be overemphasized. We assert that the very elements of the sandtray process promote play, which in turn promotes relationship. This is, in itself, elementally therapeutic. This should be an accepted maxim for sandtray therapists—who are by our perspective, play therapists—and is a wonderful discovery for the sandtray client.

Caplan and Caplan (1974) proposed several unique attributes of the process of play: (a) play is voluntary by nature, and in a world full of rules and requirements, play is refreshing and full of respite; (b) play is free from evaluation and judgment, thus it is safe to make mistakes without failure; (c) play encourages fantasy and the use of the imagination, enabling control without competition; (d) play increases involvement and interest; and (e) play encourages the development of self. These are unique attributes of sandtray therapy.

Brown and Vaughan (2009) expand on this, noting that:

- *Play is done for its own sake—it may even seem purposeless.* For clients who feel out of control [all clients?], a nondemanding sandtray experience is a welcome change and a chance to regain control.
- *Play is voluntary.* Even for the mandated client, the sandtray experience is invitational and promotes freedom.
- *Play has an inherent attraction.* There is a magnetic quality to activities that promote freedom and growth. Sandtray therapy and sandtray materials do this.
- *Play involves a freedom from time.* For therapy clients, slavery to time can be magnified. Play, and sandtray therapy, offers a respite from the captivity of pain and chaos.
- *Play helps diminish the consciousness of self.* All clients have a degree of self-consciousness that limits their growth. A play/sandtray experience takes the focus off of this negative self-talk and promotes positive self-awareness.

- *Play has an improvisational potential.* This can be seen in the wide variety of possible sandtray therapy applications.
- *Play develops a continuation desire.* In a world of work—therapy is certainly work—an activity that promotes a desire to reengage is powerful. Sandtray therapy has this potential.

We posit that the marriage of an expressive medium such as sand and play with the process of psychotherapy is a natural evolution. It becomes important, therefore, to bring some definition to the process.

Play therapy involves more than the application of traditional talk therapy accompanied by some type of play media. According to Landreth (2012), play therapy is defined as

> a dynamic interpersonal relationship between a child (or person of any age) and a therapist trained in play therapy procedures who provides selected play materials and facilitates the development of a safe relationship for the child (or person of any age) to fully express and explore self (feelings, thought, experiences, and behaviors) through play, the child's natural medium of communication. (p. 11)

This is a comprehensive definition that applies to the world of sandtray therapy as well.

Sandtray therapy should always involve a *dynamic interpersonal relationship.* Regardless of the theoretical approach or techniques used in the sandtray process, the creation and development of a dynamic interpersonal relationship is crucial. Kalff (1980) stressed the importance of the therapist creating a "free and protected space," noting that it is the love of the therapist that creates this space. This will be addressed further in Chapters 5 and 6. The sandtray therapist should be *trained in (sandtray) therapy procedures.* Appropriate training and supervised experience is crucial for the therapist interested in doing sandtray therapy. The ethical and responsible psychotherapist will become theoretically and practically grounded in any modality before its employment. This is particularly important in sandtray therapy. We have both encountered persons employing sandtray therapy with minimal training and experience—it is not just disappointing, it is a clinical and ethical concern. Note that reading this book alone is not considered adequate. Most mental health practitioners' ethical codes indicate competency is based in education, training, and supervision. Of course, we support ethical, competent work with clients.

We would also strongly suggest (and with our own supervisees, insist) that any sandtray therapist also have the experience of being a sandtray therapy client. We are obviously convinced of the power of this expressive modality—and since the personal and professional process of growth for therapists is a lifelong process—it is only appropriate that sandtray therapists experience the intra- and inter-personally evocative nature of sandtray therapy. We have both done personal work in our own trays (there's nothing quite like creating your own tray after a challenging day!), and have benefitted from the experience of being sandtray therapy clients with qualified colleagues. Additionally, it is recommended to consider therapy from sandtray therapists who practice from different theoretical approaches

As with any play therapy modality, it is crucial to *provide selected play materials* in the sandtray therapy process, as will be described in Chapter 4. A random collection of sandtray materials and miniature figures is not appropriate; an intentional and deliberate selection is. Clients may be confused by a disorganized collection, emotionally flooded by an overwhelmingly large collection, or confined by a limited collection. The collection of miniature figures should be a natural outgrowth of the sandtray therapist's training and evolving experience.

The sandtray therapist should *facilitate*, rather than direct, the therapeutic experience—even with directive interventions. Children, individuals, and families enter into the therapy process already feeling disempowered and out of control. As the sandtray therapist facilitates rather than wholly choreographs the process, clients will experience healing through a growing sense of self-control, empowerment, and safety. Siegelman (1990) described this facilitation process well:

> To be a participant-observer at the moment when a frightened or constricted patient feels securely enough held to take her first step into the realm of symbolic play—this is being a midwife to the birth of the capacity for meaning. (p. 175)

This facilitation creates the *safety* that Landreth (2012) refers to in his play therapy definition. This is reflective of Kalff's (1980) previously noted "free and protected" space. We would argue that, both inside and outside of therapy, people do not grow where they do not feel safe. Safety, a priority for any sandtray therapist, creates the avenue for change.

This safety in turns creates the opportunity for clients to *fully express and explore the self.* Self-expression and self-exploration are crucial in the counseling process, and are foundational in sandtray therapy. Kalff (1981) stressed this exploration of self: "the patient, through the sandplay, penetrates to that which we can recognize as an expression of Self" (p. viii).

Finally, the last element of Landreth's definition particularly applies to the sandtray therapy process. Play is more than just a child's *natural medium of communication.* In fact, it is a mistake to assume that cognitive verbalization and discussion are the clients' natural medium of communication, regardless of their developmental level. As suggested above, we would assert that the natural medium of communication for many clients in crisis involves some type of expressive medium.

An additional point should be made—play therapy and sandtray therapy are often thought to be treatment modalities for the individual client. We assert, however, that sandtray therapy with couples, families, and groups is both exciting and effective. This is further discussed in Chapters 8 and 9.

In fact, the marriage of family therapy and sandtray therapy is a natural union. Eliana Gil (1994) posited:

> Family therapists and play therapists share a noble trait: They are by far the most creative and dynamic therapists in existence. Family therapists . . . engage the family's participation in a dynamic way, either by intensifying or replacing verbal communication. (p. 34)

Family therapy that does *not* actively and intentionally provide a means to include children, such as an expressive media like sandtray therapy, is not truly *family* therapy. While a systemic approach to treating families is frequently preached and lauded, the exclusion of children from the process barely makes the treatment systemic. Nathan Ackerman (1970), one of the pioneers in the field, wrote "without engaging the children in a meaningful interchange across the generations, there can be no family therapy" (p. 403). Sandtray therapy creates a bridge for meaningful interchanges to take place. The content of sandtray therapy provides a metaphorical blueprint of family alliances, personality stages, and intergenerational patterns. As a largely undefended mode of expression, sandtray therapy, like art therapy, provides the therapist with the opportunity to access information that might not be verbally disclosed, as well as the opportunity to observe the family's emotional climate (Kwiatkowska, 1978).

Sandtray therapy as an expressive and projective mode of psychotherapy involving the unfolding and processing of intra- and inter-personal issues through the use of specific sandtray materials as a nonverbal medium of communication, led by the client or therapist and facilitated by a trained therapist.

SANDTRAY THERAPY DEFINED

There are numerous theoretical approaches to the therapeutic use of a collection of miniature figures and a sand tray. As mentioned earlier, we consider sandtray therapy to be cross-theoretical—as such, our definition does not include theory-specific language. Recognizing that we take a generally integrative approach to the modality, we would define sandtray therapy as follows: an expressive and projective mode of psychotherapy involving the unfolding and processing of intra- and inter-personal issues through the use of specific sandtray materials as a nonverbal medium of communication, led by the client or therapist and facilitated by a trained therapist. It is a process that seeks to promote safety and control for the client so that emotionally charged issues can be addressed through the medium.

A primary goal in sandtray therapy is to fundamentally help the client process the presenting issue—nonverbally or verbally—with sandtray therapy as the processing tool or approach. Thus, this takes priority over—but not to the exclusion of—an initial focus on meaning, insight, or cognitive restructuring. These may be important, but the client's life must become tolerable and manageable before deeper issues can be explored and processed. For us, an elementary initial goal is to provide clients with a safe, reparative, and relational experience. Our encompassing therapeutic effort, therefore, is to be fellow sojourners on the client's journey, and thus witnesses to their unique story as it unfolds in the sandtray process.

We have made the deliberate choice to use the term *sandtray therapy* in this manual. It is appropriate to distinguish our approach to the therapeutic use of sand and sandtray materials from the term *sandplay*. Sandplay specifically refers to a therapeutic sandtray approach developed by Dora Kalff (1980), the Swiss Jungian analyst who adopted this term for her approach to the modality. A brief look at Kalff and the development of sandtray therapy will be offered in the following chapter. It has been our experience that the term *sandplay* has often been used generically when referring to a wide variety of therapeutic uses of sand, a tray, miniature figures, but it is more appropriate to refer to sandplay when discussing the Jungian approach stemming from Kalff's work.

As we've asserted, sandtray therapy can be used with children, adolescents, and adults, and with individuals, groups, couples, and families. As with any therapeutic modality, its use should be with purpose and intent, and part of a professional and reasonable treatment plan. We would advise, encourage, and request that interested clinicians seek appropriate training and supervised experience in the course of employing this effective medium.

BEFORE MOVING ON . . .

Therapist preference or other client differences may lead the counselor to use sandtray therapy. Clients of all ages may be more verbal, others not as much. (Note, however, that some verbal clients may use words as a way to defend or avoid.) Some clients may be drawn to the visual, creative nature of building in the sand, just as they might be drawn to other creative art techniques. There needs to be an awareness and sensitivity on the part of the counselor, who can then provide a more effective means of communication and depth of session content than the verbal approach alone. We have often sat in our dual sandtray/talk therapy room (sandtray shelves and tray in one corner, upholstered chair and loveseat in the other) and observed adult clients looking curiously and sometimes longingly at the miniatures. Those clients almost always engage with the sandtray therapy process quickly and effectively. The experienced sandtray therapist should also be able to encourage clients who are reticent about an unfamiliar intervention. Matching the therapeutic medium with the client serves to establish the therapeutic relationship.

We've argued that sandtray is adaptive and flexible, and that it's intrapsychic and interpersonal nature touches clients in profound ways. As it is truly cross-theoretical, almost any approach or treatment technique can be adapted for use in sandtray therapy. Having made these assertions, we would emphasize that clients are not healed through the use of techniques: Clients experience healing through process and relationship. We look forward to exploring the role of sandtray therapy as a core process and relational tool in the balance of this book.

2

Some History and Rationale

Nearly as long as there has been psychotherapy, play therapy has assisted in meeting the mental health needs of children. As the field grew, the use of play as therapy expanded to adolescents, adults, couples, and families. Within the play therapy movement, sandtray therapy utilized play in another format to provide clients additional method to express and resolve their emotional and psychological pain. Through the use of the materials including a sand tray and miniature figures, clients non-verbally express that which is too painful to articulate. We are convinced not only of its efficacy as an intervention, but of its quality as a place of retreat for clients in pain. We will discuss the history of sandtray therapy and then list several rationales that include practical benefits for the use of sandtray therapy with adults, children, couples, and families.

> I set myself as a goal to work out an apparatus which would put into the child's hand a means of directly expressing his ideas and emotions, one which would allow the recording of his creations and abstracting them for study (Lowenfeld, 1979a, p. 3).

A BRIEF HISTORY

With a collection of small toy figures and trays filled with sand, Margaret Lowenfeld (1979b) began her journey of developing a mental health intervention for children: *The World Technique*. The context of the development of this new form of play therapy has always intrigued us. The Russo-Polish War in Eastern Europe in the 1920's found Lowenfeld, a London medical doctor and pediatrician, providing medical services for those experiencing the typhus outbreak and those in prisoner of war camps in Poland (1993). Alongside that work she was also a relief worker for thousands of Polish students suffering from the aftermath of the war. Returning to London, Lowenfeld observed children with the same "expressions, postures and gestures that resembled those with which I had become familiar in prison camps and famine areas" (1993, p. 2). These intense experiences impelled her to discover a method to promote the mental health issues of children, a way to allow children to share their inner worlds. Recalling the book *Floor Games* (Wells, 1911), which she had read as a young woman, and aware of the developmental limitations of children, when she opened the Clinic for Nervous and Difficult Children in October of 1928, it was complete with trays of sand and a collection of small toys (Lowenfeld, 1993). Lowenfeld stated that in less than 3 months after a metal tray with sand placed on a table and a cabinet with drawers containing miniature objects were included in the playroom, "a spontaneous new technique was developed, *created by the children themselves*" (1993, pp. 280–281). The term *World* first appeared in case notes in June of 1929 (Lowenfeld, 1993, p. 280) and continued to be commonly used by staff in case notes and case discussions. The World Technique was named.

Play therapy was concurrently being developed and utilized, beginning with Sigmund Freud's (1909) case of Little Hans and the later work of Hermine Hug-Hellmuth (1921). Anna Freud's (1965) psychoanalytic form of play therapy viewed play primarily as a means of forming a solid therapeutic alliance with the child client, while Klein (1932) believed that play could be used as a substitute for verbalization, replacing the psychoanalytic technique of free association. In a letter to The British Medical Journal in

1938, Lowenfeld and Duke clarified that there are "two clearly formulated methods of play therapy, each with its own history and technique" (p. 1281) referring to her own work and that of Melanie Klein. In this letter, Lowenfeld clearly articulates her work as play therapy and those she trained as *play therapists*. Like many of us today, she rues that too often play therapy publications do not clearly identify the specific formulation or techniques, making comparisons difficult.

Working with children in the sand tray was expanded and popularized by the work of Dora Kalff, a Swiss Jungian analyst. Kalff (2003) learned of Lowenfeld's work, studied with her in London in 1956, and adapted the method, calling the approach *Sandplay* to clearly differentiate it from the World Technique. As noted in Chapter 1, the term *sandplay* continues to identify the Jungian approach, although it has been widely used outside of Jungian circles. Kalff (1971) acknowledged Lowenfeld's important contribution: "She understood completely the child's world and created with ingenious intuition a way which enables the child to build a world—his world—in a sandbox" (p. 32).

It is interesting to note in the broader field of play therapy, Lowenfeld and Kalff are rarely mentioned in the historical timeline of the developing field. Sandtray therapy certainly is a play therapy approach, and we would put forward that the pioneers in sandtray therapy deserve recognition within the broader view of play therapy.

There are many approaches and nuances in both the theoretical and technical approaches to working with clients in the sand, ranging from the traditional Lowenfeld approach and Jungian sandplay to Gestalt methods and cognitive-behavioral approaches. Each of these (and others) has their own inherent therapeutic value. This is not surprising, even historically from Lowenfeld's perspective: Lowenfeld stated clinicians would see in any created World "components and constructs that support their views," not as "merely a result of wish fulfillment" on the part of the therapist, but "because they are almost certainly to be present there" (1993, p. 7). This was recently demonstrated by Eberts and Homeyer (2015) through processing a single creation in the sand from both a Gestalt and Adlerian perspective. More details on how to use sandtray therapy from various theoretical viewpoints in Chapter 7.

Both of us are therapists and counselor educators. If we can put on our professor caps for a moment, we'd like to make a comment about counseling theory. As educators, you would expect that we value theory, which is certainly the case. However, we would argue for being theoretically based, not theoretically bound. One can use a variety of techniques, in other words, be technically eclectic. We have concerns, however, about being theoretically eclectic.

As already noted, theory alone is inadequate—in fact, theory without technique is merely philosophy. The opposite is an equally important concern. Techniques without theory are reckless, perhaps even dangerous. (Okay—off with the professor caps.) Therefore, we strongly encourage the interested reader to seek ongoing training and supervision in sandtray therapy within an approach that resonates personally and theoretically.

WHY USE SANDTRAY THERAPY? A RATIONALE

As experienced sandtray therapists will attest, there are many benefits for both clients and counselors. Similar to other expressive and projective treatment modalities, sandtray therapy provides an important medium to reach hurting clients. We would therefore like to summarize some of the primary rationales and benefits for using sandtray therapy.

1. *Sandtray therapy gives expression to nonverbalized emotional issues.* Since play is the language of childhood, as well as a language for a client of any age who is unable or unwilling to verbalize, the sand tray provides a safe medium for expression. If play is the language, then the miniatures are the

words (adapted from Haim Ginott's famous statement). Just as an empty canvas provides a place for the artist's expression, so the tray provides a place for the client's emotional expression. The client needs no creative or artistic ability since the medium provides an experience that is free from evaluation.

The self-directed sand tray process allows clients to be fully themselves. Through the process of sandtray therapy, which includes a caring, accepting, and attuned relationship-children, adults, and families can express their total personality. This enables hurting clients to consider new possibilities, some of which are not possible through verbal expression, and thus significantly develop the expression of self. Sandtray therapy is, therefore, more than a symbolization of the psyche—it is a forum for full self-expression and self-exploration.

2. *Sandtray therapy has a unique kinesthetic quality.* We have already reflected on the sensory quality of sand and play, and the need for a sensory experience for clients in distress or crisis. Sandtray therapy provides this sensory experience, and meets the need that we all (not just our clients) have for kinesthetic experiences. This fundamental essential, an extension of very basic attachment needs, is met through relationship and experience. Sandtray therapy provides both of these elements for clients.

The very tactile experience of touching and manipulating the sand is a therapeutic experience in and of itself. We frequently have clients who, choosing not to speak, have done nothing more than run their fingers through the sand. This often results in the client's ability to talk about deep issues. It is as if the sensory experience with the sand causes a loosening of the tongue. There is now neurological support that this does in fact occur; more about that in Chapter 10. While this may not be the intent, or goal, of the session, it is certainly a therapeutic by-product. The manipulation of the sand and placement of the miniature figures is both safe and kinesthetically satisfying, especially for clients whose prior sensory experience was noxious. The tactile sensations which results from moving one's hand(s) through the sand can also reduce anxiety and help the client self-regulate. The agitated lower brain can be calmed through the tactile stimuli, which is interpreted by the limbic system as soothing (Badenoch, 2008).

3. *Sandtray therapy serves to create a necessary therapeutic distance for clients.* Clients or families in emotional crisis are often unable to express their pain in words, but may find expression through a medium such as sandtray therapy. It is simply easier for a traumatized client to "speak" through one of the sandtray therapy miniature figures than to directly verbalize their pain. The consistency of the medium, and the consistency of the therapist in allowing the client to direct the process, creates a place where the client establishes the degree of therapeutic distance. Children, adults, and families in sandtray therapy may experience emotional release through symbolization and sublimation, through the projection onto the tray and miniatures.

4. *The therapeutic distance that sandtray therapy provides creates a safe place for abreaction to occur.* Children and families that have experienced trauma need a therapeutic setting in which to abreact, a place where repressed issues can emerge and be relived, as well as to experience the negative emotions that are frequently attached. Abreaction, a crucial element in the treatment of trauma, finds facilitated expression.

5. *Sandtray therapy is an effective intervention for traumatized clients.* In addition to the needed safety that is provided for sandtray clients through the expressive and projective nature of the intervention, there are neurobiological effects of trauma that point to the need for nonverbal interventions. The sensory nature

of trauma may best be addressed though a sensory intervention such as sand tray and the neurobiological inhibitions on cognitive processing and verbalization point to the need for an expressive intervention. This is expanded upon in Chapter 10.

6. *Sandtray therapy with families is a truly inclusive experience.* An adult talk therapy approach to treating families is decidedly exclusive, as it fails to recognize and honor the developmental level of children in the family. Sandtray therapy with families overcomes this obstacle. Sandtray therapy creates a level playing field for every family member, giving each person the opportunity to express him or herself. Keith and Whitaker (1981) include play therapy interventions as an integral part of the family treatment process, concluding "fundamental family therapy takes place at this nonverbal level" (p. 249).

   For example, it can be very threatening and a developmental impossibility to ask a child to detail the communication patterns in the family through words. It can be equally threatening for any member of the family who feels isolated or disempowered. Put simply, it is taboo to "air the dirty laundry," especially to an outsider. Family members "aren't supposed to" talk about problems. Perhaps the sandtray therapy miniature figures can! The typical family sculpting exercise, which can be overwhelming for children to do in a family session, may be replicated in the sand tray. Like puppet play, sand tray play can create "an unrealistic and nonthreatening atmosphere that assists in the identification process, thereby encouraging the projection of emotional aspects and interpersonal relationships through the characters" (Bow, 1993, p. 28). Chapter 9 provides specific details on working with couples and families with sandtray therapy.

7. *Sandtray therapy naturally provides boundaries and limits*, which promote safety for the client. Boundaries and limits define the therapeutic relationship. Sweeney (1997) suggested: "A relationship without boundaries is not a relationship; rather, it is an unstructured attempt at connection that cannot be made because the people have no specific rules for engagement. A world without limits is not a safe world, and children do not grow where they do not feel safe" (p. 103).

   The careful structure of the sandtray therapy process and the carefully selected tools of the sandtray therapist provide the client with the boundaries that create the sense of safety needed for growth. The size of the sand tray, the size and selection of miniature figures, the office setting, and the guidance and instruction of the therapist all provide boundaries and limits for the client. While these limits are imperative and intentional, they promote freedom for expression. These inherent limits to sandtray therapy bring a focus to the therapeutic process, which in addition to promoting the safety which boundaries bring, assist the client to focus on the therapeutic issues to be addressed.

8. *Sandtray therapy provides a unique setting for the emergence of therapeutic metaphors.* There is an increasing amount of literature on metaphors and psychotherapy, much of which focuses on verbal metaphors. Siegelman (1990) suggested that metaphors "combine the abstract and the concrete in a special way, enabling us to go from the known and the sensed to the unknown, and the symbolic. . . . They achieve this combination in a way that typically arises from and produces strong feeling that leads to integrating insight" (p. ix). Metaphors can indeed be therapeutically powerful. We would suggest that the most powerful metaphors in therapy are those that are generated by the clients themselves. Sandtray therapy creates a consummate setting for this to occur. The sand and miniatures are ideal for clients to express their own therapeutic

metaphors. Clients often express that they don't know what one or more min-iature figures initially means to them or why they selected it, but that it 'just needs to be there'. The ability of a client to release the need to build a logical, sequential, literal, left-brained scene, results in the use of symbols, imagery, and feelings that are right-brained. When clients choose to remain intuitive, and respond with a more right-brained action, meaningful symbols and meta-phors are formed in the tray.

Where therapeutic metaphors emerge, therapeutic interpretation naturally follows. We would echo Kalff's (1980) warning against focusing on interpreta-tion, recognizing that it is the client's interpretation that is the most important. We would further suggest that interpretation of sandtrays is not essential to the healing process, and often need to remind ourselves that when we interpret, we do so with our own minds and experiences, not the client's. It is a helpful reminder that when interpreting a client's expression of an experience that the sharing of the interpretation is meant to serve the needs of the client, and not the curiosity of the therapist.

9. *Sandtray therapy is effective in overcoming client resistance.* It is important to remember when working with children and families, that involuntary clients are frequent and typical. Children generally do not self-refer, and not all family members are enthusiastic about entering therapy. Sandtray therapy, because of its nonthreatening and engaging qualities, can captivate the involuntary cli-ent and draw in the reticent family member. Since play is the natural medium of communication for children, child clients who have been compelled into therapy by an adult are generally amenable to treatment because they are being allowed to express self through the familiar activity of play.

For the resistant adult or family member, sandtray therapy provides a means of communicating that diverts away from the fear of verbal conflict. With cou-ples, for example, it is not unusual for one partner to be less enthusiastic or even reluctant to participate. Related to this, the level of contribution that each fam-ily member makes to the construction of the sand tray scene may be a reflec-tion of the level of his or her investment in the family. In this regard, resistance can be overcome by participation in sandtray therapy, and it can be more fully identified as well.

10. *Sandtray therapy provides a needed and effective communication medium for the client with poor verbal skills.* Beyond the developmental importance of providing children with a nonverbal therapeutic medium, there are clients of all ages who have poor verbal skills, for a variety of reasons. Poor verbal skills include clients who experience developmental language delays or deficits, cli-ents with social or relational difficulties, clients with physiological challenges, and more. This includes clients who use English as a second language. Many bilingual clients prefer to express themselves in counseling in their first lan-guage. Sandtray therapy allows for the expression of deep and personal issues in a common, symbolic language.

Just as the toddler who wants something desperately but cannot commu-nicate this to the parent, so anyone can have a high level of frustration when unable to effectively communicate needs. When the toddler has a tantrum because he cannot communicate his want or need, there is an intense relation-ship challenge between parent and child. In the same way, many types of rela-tionship challenges emerge in families when family members are not able to verbalize their wants and needs. The sandtray therapy process creates a place where expression of needs and wants is not dependent upon words. The client with poor verbal skills, regardless of its etiology, finds a place of relief in the sand tray—a place where expression does not depend upon verbal acuity, but on the freedom of the medium.

11. *Conversely, sandtray therapy cuts through verbalization used as a defense.* For the pseudo-mature child who presents as verbally astute yet is developmentally unable to effectively communicate on a cognitive level, sandtray therapy provides a means to communicate through the child's true and natural medium of communication. For the verbally sophisticated adult, who uses intellectualization, rationalization, or storytelling as a defense, sandtray therapy may cut through these defenses. This is an important dynamic to be aware of, since a family system that includes a verbally well-defended member may also include one or more members unable to establish effective communication and relationship. The nonverbal and expressive nature of working in the sand tray identifies this dynamic and provides a way to address it.

12. *Sandtray therapy creates a place for child, adult, couple, family, or group clients to experience control.* One of the primary results of crisis and trauma is a loss of control for those involved. The loss of emotional, psychological, and even physiological control is one of the most distressing results. Both the individual and family in crisis feel the frustration and fear of having lost control. A crucial goal for these clients must be to re-empower them.

    The self-directed process of sandtray therapy creates a place for control to be returned. For the client looking to attain and extend self-control, sandtray therapy establishes the boundaries and allows the freedom for this to occur. For the client attempting to avoid responsibility, the sand tray process places the responsibility for and control of the process on the client. If a goal of therapy is to help clients achieve a greater internal locus of control, sandtray therapy is an effective means toward this end. The selection of a miniature figure to symbolize a trauma or other distressing event can provide the client a way to concretize it, providing emotional and psychological control and power over it.

13. *The challenge of transference may be effectively addressed through sandtray therapy.* The presence of an expressive medium creates an alternative object of transference. Lowenfeld (1979a) proposed that in the creation of worlds in the sand, transference occurred between the client and the tray, rather than between client and therapist. Weinrib (1983) noted that the sand tray often becomes an independent object, so that the client may take away images of the tray rather than an image of the therapist. Regardless of one's theoretical view of transference, however, sandtray therapy provides a means for transference issues to be safely addressed as needed. The tray and miniature figures may become objects of transference, or the means by which transference issues are safely addressed.

14. *Lastly, deeper intrapsychic issues may be accessed more thoroughly and more rapidly through sandtray therapy.* Helping a client to access underlying emotional issues and unconscious conflicts is a challenge for any counselor.

    Although certainly not a comprehensive list, the qualities of sandtray therapy that have been suggested generate an atmosphere where deep and complex intrapsychic issues can be safely approached. Most clients have some level of motivation to change, as reflected by their presence in psychotherapy. Most of these clients likewise are often well defended when confronting challenges to their ego, which has already been injured. Sandtray therapy serves to decrease ego controls and other defenses and foster greater levels of disclosure. This in turn creates an increased capacity to consider interpersonal and intrapersonal alternatives.

Bonnie Badenoch (2008) discussed the broader perspective of sandtray therapy and the brain. Badenoch indicated that use of a sand tray awakens and regulates the right-brain limbic processes, promoting vertical integration in the right brain. New neural pathway "templates" are developed, effectively rewiring dysfunctional painful memories. Badenoch indicates that touching the sand activates the brain. The sensations travel to the prefrontal cortex, which makes sense of tactile input. The counselor and client stay attuned during the building of the tray, according to Badenoch, through right-brain resonance. Additionally, "[w]hen the client recalls painful experiences and is met with empathy and kindness, new synapses carry that information throughout the brain, and blood flow changes course to more soothing paths" (p. 12). Once the tray, or world, is created, verbally discussing the content results in left and right brain integration. Adding words to the story, which occurs in the left brain, to the imagery and feelings of the right brain, strengthens and grows the corpus callosum (the connecting tissue between the left and right brain hemispheres) resulting in greater regulation of the emotional content of the sandtray experience. Badenoch indicates that the use of the miniatures as symbols, even without the use of the sand, but with verbal conversation, also stimulates this bilateral integration, thus developing the regulating experience (p. 227). "Grounded in the body, sandplay unfolds through the limbic region and cortex, and spans both hemispheres as the symbolic unfolds into words" (p. 220).

SOME FINAL THOUGHTS

There are myriads of techniques used and advocated in the mental health profession. Hurting people, however, are not healed through technique. People experience emotional healing when they encounter someone and when they encounter self. It is an inner process, a relational process, and a heart process. King Solomon suggested, "Keep thy heart with all diligence; for out of it are the issues of life" (Proverbs 4:23). Verbal therapies that keep the focus on cognitive issues don't consider the importance of the heart, which bring to us the issues of life. We submit that sandtray therapy is more than just another cross-theoretical treatment modality, because sandtray therapy seeks and maintains this inner core. Spare (1981) wrote: "As with every aspect of clinical practice, meaningful use of sandtray therapy is a function of our own human hearts, and of the ever ongoing interplay between our own centers and the centers, hearts, and needs of those we are privileged to see in psychotherapy" (p. 208).

> Learn your theories as well as you can, but put them aside, when you touch the miracle of the living soul (Jung, 1928, p. 361).

3

Sand and the Sand Tray

In this and the following chapter, we will discuss the materials which are necessary for sandtray therapy: sand and a sand tray (this chapter); miniature figures and a therapeutic space (Chapter 4). It seems quite straightforward, a rectangular box partially filled with sand. However, it is important to take a look at these essential elements and their inherent philosophical significance and importance to the client and therapeutic process. We will also comment on the availability and use of water for the sandtray therapy experience. Finally, we will provide a discussion regarding the color blue coating the inside of the tray.

THE SAND

Sand is the basic medium for this engrossing and effective treatment modality. It is a basic elemental compound, one of the most simple and common on Earth. The choice to use sand as the foundation for sandtray therapy was not accidental, but is rather a natural phenomenon. The Old Testament tells us that "the Lord God formed man of the dust of the ground, and breathed into his nostrils the breath of life" (Genesis 2:7). Our connection to this Earth is foundational. This is not accidental, but rather providential design. As we connect with the sand, we cannot help but feel the connection to the spirit within, and the Creation without (Sweeney, 1999).

Sand is also a reminder of history. A single grain of sand may have traveled thousands of miles and an equal number of years before coming to its current place of rest. Geology reminds us that a "grain was produced by forces that made the rock it was eroded from, by the Earth's surface environment that eroded it from its parent and carried it to a resting place, and by the internal deformation of the Earth's crust that buried it" (Siever, 1988, p. 1). People have had much the same experience. Many forces have come to bear on every person; some from the family of origin, some from other socio-environmental factors, some from immersion in the technological/information age, and some from crisis and trauma. The "internal deformation" of a grain of sand speaks metaphorically of the intrapsychic pain that many of our clients bring to us. Sand is a product of its history, and so are we (Sweeney, 1999).

While many factors are involved, it is because of this—this core, this essence, and this foundational element of sand—that sandtray therapy can be so impacting. Therapeutic connection and processing of rooted emotional turmoil are not merely assisted by the use of sand. It is the sand that creates the path. Eichoff (1952) suggested that sand was the "means of which gross feelings can be expressed, for it can be thrown, tossed, molded, plastered, dug and smoothed; and on this base concrete symbol can be placed . . ." (p. 235). Sand is more than a therapeutic medium. It is a means of expressing the very core of who we are. Indeed, as Dora Kalff (1981) so succinctly stated: "The act of playing in the sand allows the patient to come near his own totality" (p. vii).

Sand and play naturally relate with each other. Children and adults delight in playing in the sand at the ocean's edge, and making sandcastles—testimonies not only to their creative abilities but also expressions of themselves. In Eastern and Native-American cultures, sand is often used ritualistically. In Western culture, we hear about the sand-man helping children to get to sleep. Sand has been equated with grit or courage, as Mark Twain talks about having "sand in his craw." Sand is used in the hourglass to mark the passing of time. Sand has an ethos of its own, and as such has a basic therapeutic quality.

Early developers and researchers at the same time as Lowenfeld may or may not have actually used sand. Some, like Erikson (Homburger, 1938), used a designated area on a table, with no sand or tray. Albion used a round tray while Kamp and Kessler used a table with a rounded end and neither had sand (cited in Bradway, Signell, Spare, Stewart, Stewart, & Thompson, 1981, pp. 11–12). Bühler (1951a, 1951b) ran the first studies on Lowenfeld's technique. She used a variety of options, sandbox, floor space, or table. She indicated the English and Norwegian children had access to sandboxes, and so provided them a choice; conversely, Dutch children had only access to floor or table space.

A current sandtray therapist, working with U.S. veterans who served in the Middle East, uses no sand. She indicates for these clients, sand is therapeutically counterproductive. Another sandtray therapist recently shared regarding her final session with a client:

> her work in the sand seems so significant to her. I observed that it seemed very satisfying to work in the sand and that several times I had seen her "lean on" or "push" into the sand. These simple observations by me led her to discuss what it was like for her to work in the sand and how she "needed it," especially today." She also indicated that her client, unlike previous sessions, placed no objects in the sand tray, the client wanted to terminate her work only with the sand.

SAND TYPES AND ALTERNATIVES

There are various types of sand that can be used in the tray. We generally use generic, inexpensive play sand, which can be purchased from many major home and building outlet stores or lumberyards. This sand, which typically comes in 50-pound bags, is normally sterilized and usually free of pebbles. Sand from the beach may be used, but cannot be guaranteed to be free of contaminants. If beach sand is used, it needs several washings using clear water to remove any lingering sea-life. While the consistency of the sand is determined by the therapist, we would recommend sand that is not too coarse, which is often filled with small pebbles; or too fine, which may create dust and allergy problems because it is ground so finely that it is close to a powder. One sand vendor offers 'river bed' sand. Described as 'smooth grains and crunchy texture' it is much coarser than what one might typically use. However, I (Linda) have a student who vastly prefers the river bed sand option. Other students shun it. The point being that there are several options, and selecting the one which appeals to you is fine; but ones you shun might be just the option chosen by some clients.

Some therapists additionally choose colored sand as alternatives for clients. We have secondary trays with colored sand and find many clients enjoy the change of texture and different hues of sand. Some options are naturally occurring white and terra cotta colored sands; white 'sand' made of ground glass; or the red-purple of ground garnet. These are specifically marketed to sandtray and play therapists. Other artificially colored sands can be found in arts and crafts stores, labeled as "art sand". One elementary student recently informed his school counselor that having sand in the colors of the emotions from the movie, Inside Out, would really "help other kids work on their feelings."

A primary consideration in all these options, however, is that some clients simply view sand as needing to be the natural beige or light brown, and are alienated by colored sand. Additionally, consider the inherent importance of being 'grounded' in the sand in the tray—then naturally occurring 'real' sand would philosophically be the 'sand' of choice.

While we clearly support the use of sand for this treatment modality, there are circumstances that dictate the use of another material in the tray. We encourage therapists to carefully consider what would be most effective in their setting, keeping in mind not only clinical issues, but professional and business concerns as well.

Some therapists hold sandtray therapy sessions in carpeted rooms, and find that clean-up of spilled sand is quite challenging. Having a hand-vacuum for a quick clean-up between sessions is helpful. Then regular vacuuming with a larger unit usually takes care of the inevitable spilled sand. We have also seen the use of rice and corn meal as alternatives, which are often easier to vacuum in case of spilling. Also, if working with very small children or mentally-challenged individuals who might potentially eat the tray contents, corn meal may be a safe alternative. A limitation of these food materials, however, is that water obviously cannot be added without quite a mess occurring. Another consideration might be the clinical setting where sterility and hygiene are major concerns, such as in a hospital. Small glass or plastic beads, which can be sterilized, may be an acceptable alternative. All of these provide a varying sensory experience.

We do believe that the sand (or alternative material) is key to the therapeutic process. Placing miniature figures on a flat surface minimizes the therapeutic effect. As we have noted, the mere manipulation of the sand has therapeutic value. The sensory experience of manipulating the sand as well as placing figures in the sand is fundamental to the processing of intrapsychic issues, which are also sensory in nature.

THE SAND TRAY

The tray is more than merely a container for the sand. It is a container of the psyche as well. Jung (1977) talked about the concept of *temenos*. *Temenos* is a Greek word meaning the sacred space surrounding a temple or an altar. Jung used the word to describe a deep inner space within people where *soul-making* occurs. *Temenos* speaks of a boundary between what is sacred and what is profane. For Jung, the therapy experience was one of *temenos*. This is not only true of the sandtray therapy process, but also the sand tray itself. The tray is a container of the psyche, and involves *temenos*, where the sacred is kept separate from the profane.

The selection or construction of a tray should therefore be as deliberate and intentional as the selection of the miniature figures. There are many possibilities; we will talk about some general guidelines and what we typically use.

Lowenfeld's (1991) tray measured 27 inches by 18 inches and 1¾ inches deep. It was wooden and lined with zinc, making it waterproof. Today, the 'standard' is a rectangular tray approximately 30 inches by 20 inches, and 3 inches deep (see Figure 3.1) which is close to the Dora Kalff dimensions. These can be constructed or purchased (see Appendix B for resources), and are usually made of wood or plastic. It is recommended that the tray be waterproof, which is usually accomplished by paint or a waterproof finish.

It is certainly possible to have a tray that is in another shape, such as square, round, or octagonal—but what is more important is the overall size. Just as the collection of miniature figures should not be too large and thus overwhelming, the sand tray needs to be psychologically and practically manageable as well. A primary issue here is that it is more therapeutically effective to have a sand tray that can be viewed and visually examined in a single glance, without having to move the eyes or head to observe all parts of the creation. This is important for both the client(s) and therapist. It visually, as well as physically, contains. The entire creation in the sand is then able to be 'taken in' as one scene, or gestalt, defined as "something that is made of many parts and yet is

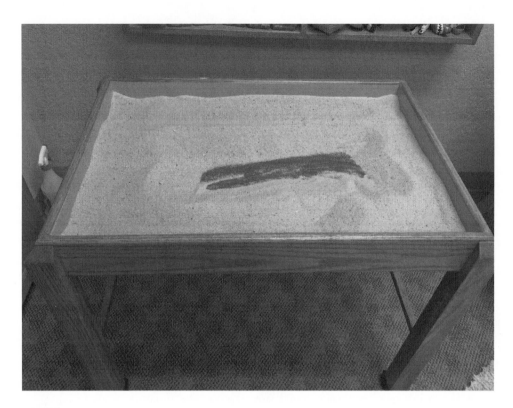

FIGURE 3.1 Standard sand tray

somehow more than or different from the combination of its parts" (Merriam-Webster). This provides the possibility of client integration and movement from a part to a greater whole. An exception to the size is when one uses a larger tray for group or family work. That will be addressed in later chapters.

Some therapists prefer to use round trays, as they may lend themselves to the creation of a *mandala* (a Sanskrit word meaning "circle"). Mandalas have significant meaning in some spiritual settings. Carl Jung viewed mandalas as representations of the unconscious self, and that the creating of them helps move the client toward greater wholeness. The shape of the tray, therefore, may be related to the therapist's theoretical orientation or personal preference. Round trays can be purchased from specialized vendors (see Appendix B). Also, plant saucers of various sizes may provide a variety of options (see Figure 3.2).

Other options for sand trays are the small, restaurant take-out containers for use by large groups of people, such as classroom guidance experiences (see Figure 3.3). We have also used the smaller plant saucers for similar large group experiences where individual trays were desired.

Many clients need the additional boundaries created by the size and structure of the container. As the client creates a world or picture scene, both the therapist and client are able to behold and consider the unfolding of the psyche in a comprehensive view. (Those clients with high boundary and containing needs will also use fences and other containers within the container offered by the tray itself; more on that later.) Also, since it is recommended to take a photograph of the completed scene in the sandtray for record keeping, consultation, and processing with the client, the quality of the photographic record decreases if the tray is too large.

Some final comments on the size and shape of the tray: We have found the standard size and shape to be generally advantageous for several reasons. A tray that is smaller may be too confining and may limit a fuller expression of self for the client. A tray that

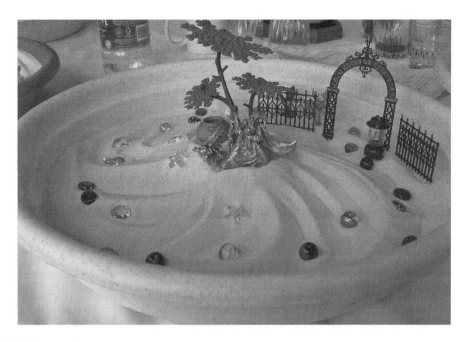

FIGURE 3.2   Plant saucer as sand tray

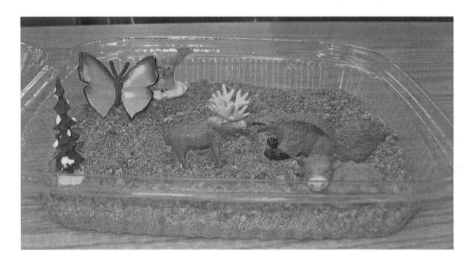

FIGURE 3.3   Take-out box as sand tray

is larger may be too expansive and thus overwhelming for the client and the psyche. The rectangular shape facilitates dividing the sandtray scene into sections; noting that clients often need to separate and compartmentalize issues. In contrast, a round tray provides no ready corners in which to facilitate this compartmentalization, or to "hide" if necessary. Conversely, the round tray may promote the formation of the mandala or centering of the self.

Manufactured sand trays may be too costly and cumbersome for some clinical situations. While it is important that the therapist provide the materials for the medium, it is equally important that the therapist maintain an affordable (and occasionally, transportable) clinical setting. An alternative tray that we have used is a clear plastic sweater box, with a blue lid that can serve as both a cover and be slid underneath the tray to create the recommended blue tray bottom.

The placement of the sand tray is also a point of consideration. We generally recommend that the tray be no higher than the usual table height, a comfortable level for most people. The height should certainly reflect and accommodate the height of the client, recognizing the range from small children to adults. We favor the placement of the tray on a portable cart. In addition to flexibility in terms of the storage of materials, a portable cart gives the client the opportunity to walk around the tray when pondering scenes and placing miniature figures.

It is also helpful to have the tray sit on a surface where several inches of surface space are available around the perimeter of the tray. Some clients like to place miniature figures outside of the tray or bridge scenes from the outside to the inside of the tray. This may be a reflection of therapeutic issues that clients aren't able or willing to address yet, or representative of boundaries that clients are creating regarding people or circumstances that they do not want in their lives.

And finally, Daniel has used trays with a 1 to 2 inch lip around the top of the tray sides. This can facilitate placing figures on the lip, above the sand. Linda has had clients line up some images along the inner side of the tray, and believes if the tray had a lip, those items would have indeed been placed above the created scene within the tray, while still remaining part of the creation.

WET AND DRY SAND AND SAND TRAYS

We strongly recommend having two trays available, one wet and the other dry. There are distinct advantages to having water available for the client who needs to mold and shape the sand. Some clients simply prefer to work in damp sand. However, if only one tray is available and excessive water is used the tray may remain too wet, thus unusable by future clients that day. If a client uses a great deal of water, the sand may need a day or two to dry. A hint on quick drying: Form a large mountain or pyramid in the tray. This increases the surface area and the sand usually dries sufficiently overnight.

Children in particular may want to have oceanic-wet experiences. For occasions such as this, a deep plastic container works. It's easier to allow lots of water knowing when the session is done the standing water can be poured off.

Another method, taught to us by middle school students, is to place containers into the sand, and fill those with water. The containers varied from blue plastic-foam boxes (which once held mushrooms), to small, clear condiment cups. This resulted in a creative way to contain water within the tray, providing both another container and a volume of water.

Like sand, water has a unique sensory and kinesthetic quality that touches the psyche at a deep level. It may symbolize cleansing and rebirth or flooding and death, or any number of metaphors. Water changes the consistency and malleability of the sand. Margaret Lowenfeld (1967) commented upon this:

> Sand and water lend themselves to the demonstration of a large variety of fantasies, as for example, tunnel making, burying or drowning, land and seascapes. When wet, the sand may be molded, and when dry it is pleasant to feel, and many tactile experiments can be made with the gradual addition of moisture. Wet sand can be dried up again and reconverted to wet, or by adding further water it becomes "slosh," and finally water when the dry land has completely disappeared. (pp. 47–48)

One possible way to set up the duo of a wet and dry tray is to have both on a mobile cart, with the dry tray on top. The second tray—the wet tray—can be in a plastic tray, like the clear plastic sweater box mentioned above. When the client wishes to use the wet tray, it will fit inside or on top of the dry tray on the top of the cart, and when not used can be stored on a lower shelf.

One compromise that we have used when only one tray is available is allowing clients to use a spray bottle of water. Clients can use a minimal amount of moisture to help sculpt the sand, and the sand does not get soaked with water and is available for dry use with later clients.

THE COLOR BLUE

It is universally accepted that the inside of the tray should be blue on the bottom, to simulate water, and on the sides, to simulate sky. Steinhardt (1997), an art therapist and sandplay therapist in Israel, challenges us to look at and think further about a blue interior to the tray. A darker blue color encourages depth work, but Steinhardt cautions against the use of too dark a hue, which can bring on grief responses. Equally, too light a shade of blue for the sky-line on the sides of the tray may have the effect of no longer containing the work within the tray. According to Walkes (cited in Steinhardt, 1997), the color blue triggers neurotransmitters which calm the entire body; lower blood pressure, providing the ability to handle threatening material; slow the pulse rate and deepen breathing, eliminating the flight or fright response (p. 52). Steinhardt uses a medium cerulean-blue in her dry trays; a darker cobalt-blue in the wet tray (1997, p. 461). Linda has custom painted my primary sand tray with a darker blue on the bottom and a sky blue on the sides. Some clients appear to notice and appreciate the differences when building their worlds (Homeyer, in press).

4

Miniature Figures
Selection and Arrangement

Miniature figures are the words, symbols, and metaphors of the client's nonverbal communication. It is through the use of the miniature figures that clients are able to express feelings, thoughts, beliefs, and desires that may be too overwhelming for words. Or, more typically for the client using a sand tray, miniature figures are the symbols and metaphors that provide an expression for that which is still beyond words.

In play therapy, we believe that toys are the child's words and play is the child's language (Ginott, 1960). Sandtray therapy is similar, allowing the client to communicate through the use of miniatures and the completed creation in the sand. Therefore, it is crucial to provide the client with a diverse vocabulary. While it may be unreasonable to provide every word that the client may need (just as our talk therapy clients rarely utilize most words in the dictionary), it is incumbent upon the sandtray therapist to provide several choices from a variety of basic categories. Gisela Schubach DeDomenico (1995) writes,

> A good selection taps the imagery of life: the cosmos; the Earth; and the mineral, plant, animal, and human kingdoms. Remember you are not creating an art gallery. Nor are you creating a world of deprivation. Therefore, you need to include that which repels you, that which magnetically draws you, that which bores you, that which is tasteless, that which is horrifying, that which is good, that which is evil, that which is harmonious, that which is absurd, etc. (p. 45)

The early professional literature suggests approximately 300 miniatures be available to a client for use in a psychotherapy session (Bühler, 1951a, 1951b). Ryce-Menuhin (1992) states he has approximately 1,000 miniatures and finds this a facilitative number of choices. We have found that once we began collecting, we see and find them everywhere: Every conference, every trip, almost every outing results in returning with yet another addition to the collection. It may be a seashell from a trip to the coast, a junk and dragon from a trip to Chinatown in San Francisco, a fairyland castle from Disney World, an unusual rock from a walk, a pirate-ship from the local discount toy store—well, you get the idea. This collecting of miniature figures becomes addictive (non-clinically speaking, of course!).

There is no exact number of miniatures for the sandtray therapist to have. If you catch the 'addiction,' as we have, it is easy to build a collection that becomes too big. Obviously, a limited collection means a limited symbolic vocabulary, and can be emotionally constricting for clients. On the other side, a collection that is too large can lead to disorganization and may be emotionally flooding for clients. There is no research regarding the prime number of items for the collection, certainly it is an individual preference. However, we suggest that the decision be based on intentional decision making, not simply collecting, collecting, and collecting yet more.

Badenoch writes of the client's "ability to generate an interpersonal system with the sand and her chosen symbols . . . creating new representations of comfort and release in a visceral rather than cognitive way . . ." (2008, p. 236).

GUIDELINES FOR SELECTION

There are a few guidelines regarding the selection of miniature figures. Some are simply common sense, or theoretical in nature, and others are driven by financial considerations. Viewing the collections of colleagues, observing pictures as part of conference presentations, and brochures of those few, but specialized, sand tray vendors can expand initial thoughts and ideas.

Here are some suggestions regarding the selection of miniatures:

a. Miniature
b. Not in scale
c. Regionally sensitive
d. Natural materials

1. Generally speaking, the miniature figures should be just that, miniature.
2. However, this is not model railroading (although those stores are valuable sources) where scale is paramount. For therapeutic sand tray work it is facilitative for the items to not be in scale with one another. A client wishing to express just how overwhelming her fear is may place a 12-inch tall T-Rex dinosaur in her sandtray. Or, conversely, a client desiring to communicate how small and overlooked he feels at work may use the smallest human figure in the collection.
3. In fact, we specifically recommend a few non-miniature figures. These should be predatory animals, such as a larger-than-life spider, nearly life-sized rat, and a large (12- to 14-inch) snake, along with their miniature-sized counterparts. When clients are traumatized from abuse, the victimizer is often initially represented in the tray by a large predatory creature. The power differential between victim and victimizer is aptly represented with the large creatures.
4. The miniature figures should be representative of your client's world. Here are some suggestions to stimulate your thinking:
   a. The people, family groups to occupational, should reflect a variety of ethnicities (especially those which are representative of your clientele).
   b. Vegetation can be selected to reflect your region of the country. In Texas and the Southwest one might have a variety, from cacti to palm trees. The Pacific Northwest might have more evergreen trees.
   c. Houses also vary from single-family dwellings to apartment buildings. Buildings and structures can have a regional motif, for example, Linda (living near San Antonio) has an Alamo miniature, and Daniel (living near Portland) has a miniature Mt. Hood.
5. Miniature items are made of a variety of materials. Plastic certainly makes for more durable (generally) and inexpensive items. Initially, most of your miniatures may be plastic for this reason. However, we find natural materials to be therapeutically important. We tend to be very separated from nature and the things of the earth. To see, touch, and experience items made from natural materials (shaped, carved, or in the original form) such as wood, minerals, rock, and such, can assist the client in reconnecting. This tactile stimulus can trigger new neuropathways while in the process of building in the tray. Clients have been observed holding a figure throughout the building process. Our observation is that the figure is generally one of a natural material, or a heavy figure made of ceramic material, or one with texture, like a carved material.

Miniatures made of pewter, regardless of whether the items are people, wizards, princesses, castles, knights, gargoyles, or whatever, also have the weight and texture components. Some clients prefer the natural, unpainted figures (like carved wood) and others seem drawn to semiprecious metal. Can't afford pewter or other gold or silver items? Painting items with pewter, silver, or gold paint can take care of this. While the feel of the item is different (weight and texture), there will still be the visual advantage.

Often clients will desire to express an "otherworldly" world by using all pewter (or silver or gold). Paint is a way to offer this option without a great deal of expense.

CATEGORIES

Categories assist the sandtray therapist to select a variety of miniatures and build a balanced collection. Initially, most counselors begin a collection by selecting several miniature figures from each category. The items selected should provide as wide a representation of that category as possible. The counselor can then add to the overall collection over time.

Just as clients are drawn to certain miniature figures and items, we as sandtray therapists can also be drawn to certain types or categories. Consequently, it is important to add to our set of miniature figures in a balanced manner. We once read (source unknown) that sometimes merely looking at a collection of miniatures can tell us a lot about the collector, similar to what a creation in the tray might tell us about a client. Think about that a moment. Sure, get the miniatures that "speak to you," but add others, too, for a useful, balanced set. By the way, if you acquire a miniature that particularly speaks strongly to you, or is valuable, we suggest that you do not add it to your sandtray therapy selection. Better to keep these in your own personal tray (we both have these!). If your "favorite" miniature becomes broken, stolen, or mistreated in some way, you will respond in a way that could interrupt the therapeutic process.

Categories are also useful when setting up the arrangement of the miniature collection, but more on that later.

People

A wide variety of people are particularly useful.

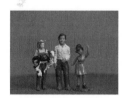

FIGURE 4.1 People

- *Family groups*—This includes adults, teenagers, children, babies, and the elderly. More than one family is necessary, given the number of step/blended/single-parent households and large extended families. A variety of ethnic figures is paramount and should reflect your clientele. It's valuable to have lots of babies—crawling, sitting, sleeping, in a high chair, in a stroller, in a baby buggy, and so on. We've also found teenagers talking on the phone have been used effectively by clients—parents as well as teens. Elderly men and women can be more difficult to locate, but worth the search.
- *Brides and grooms*—Since many relationships break-up and marriages end in divorce, it's helpful if the figures are not connected. The figures can be placed together or separately. This is especially useful for those clients working through separation and divorce issues.
- *Occupational*—This would be a variety of human figures clothed for a variety of jobs and occupations. These might be mechanics, doctors, nurses, rescue personnel, policemen, firemen, priest, clergy, sailors, soldiers, and so on. Clients often use "helpers," such as doctors, EMTs, and firemen to represent needed or wanted rescue. Judges are useful for clients involved in divorce or custody situations. Also, children in foster care often know that "the judge" controls their lives. As possible, have both genders represented and variety of ethnicities if possible (these are harder to locate). One of Linda's students recently noted that the professional figures were all Anglo; the tradesmen were minorities. While we purchase what is made easily available to us, seeking out other options, and sharing those sources, continues to assist in helping the field serve more effectively and with sensitivity.

- *Hobbies*—We have found that two figures, a man pushing a lawn mower and a woman gardening, have been used extensively by 9- to 11-year-olds. People being involved in other hobby activities can be found, such as a hunter with a rifle.
- *Sports*—Males and female figures playing sports—basketball, football, soccer, skiers, tennis players, bicyclers, and so on. Again, beginning sets might have those that pertain to one's geographic areas. For example, in Dallas, the Cowboys (football players) might be a must! If you see children and teens in your practice, you might want to have basketball and soccer figures.
- *Stage-of-life figures*—Graduates, Bar Mitzvah/Bat Mitzvah, First Communion, pregnancy, parents (adult figures holding baby/child), formal dress (prom/wedding attendants/ debutantes/quinceanera, etc.). Remember, male and female figures of each.
- *Historical figures*—This opens up a large grouping of human figures: kings, queens, knights; cave men and women; military heroes, soldiers; cowboys and Indians; astronauts; pirates; knights and other medieval characters, and so on. Daniel has a miniature Adolph Hitler—which represents hate, evil, and prejudice. Some clients are repulsed by, and others attracted to this figure.

Animals

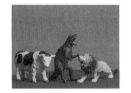

FIGURE 4.2 Animals

- *Prehistoric*—Dinosaurs are a particular must, especially if working with children.
- *Zoo/wild*—This grouping includes anything one might see at the zoo: elephants, giraffes, tigers, lions, bears (brown, polar, koala), penguins, buffalo, moose, gorillas, hippopotamuses, monkeys, alligators, crocodiles, snakes (all kinds, coiled, uncoiled).
- *Farm/domestic*—Cows, horses, sheep, goats, chickens, ducks, dogs, cats, and such. Have lots of horses—it seems that preadolescent girls use a lot of horses.
- *Birds*—Parrots, eagles, storks, peacocks, penguins, flamingos, owls, sea gulls, bird nests.
- *Insects*—Spiders, flies, roaches, caterpillars, all manner of 'creepy-crawlies'.
- *Sea life*—Whales, dolphins, sharks, octopus, various smaller fishes, clams, lobsters.

Buildings

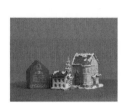

FIGURE 4.3 Buildings

- *Houses*—Single-family houses, apartment buildings, simple, ornate, huts, log cabins, adobe, burned out and damaged houses.
- *Business/civil*—Schools, firehouses, office buildings, garages, jails/prisons, gas stations, lighthouses, hospitals.
- *Religious*—Churches, pagodas, temples, mosques.
- *Historical*—Castles, forts, teepees. (We have a miniature of the World Trade Center twin towers, which obviously carries considerable meaning.)
- *Other*—Military tents, barns, and such.

Transportation

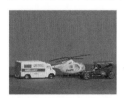

FIGURE 4.4 Transportation

- *Cars*—Typical family cars, minivans, SUVs, police cars, sports cars, antique cars, limousines, racing cars, taxis.
- *Trucks*—Military trucks, farm trucks, emergency vehicles, ambulances, rescue vehicles, dump trucks, bulldozers, buses (school/Greyhound-like), fire engines.

- *Flight vehicles*—Airliners, military planes, helicopters, jet planes, space shuttles, space rockets, spaceships.
- *Nautical*—Fishing boats, yachts, canoes, rubber rafts, ocean liners, military landing craft, submarines, rowboat.
- *Other*—Motorcycles, bicycles, train cars, covered wagon, Cinderella-type coach.

Vegetation

- *Trees*—Trees with leaves, trees without leaves, trees with autumn-colored leaves, palm trees, pine trees, Christmas trees.
- *Other*—Bushes, hedges, cacti, flowers.

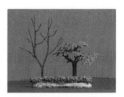

FIGURE 4.5 Vegetation

Fences/Gates/Signs

- *Fences, fences, and more fences!*—Clients tend to do a lot of fencing in and fencing out, so have plenty available. A helpful suggestion is to have enough to completely fence in the perimeter of your tray, with some left over. Sometimes fences come in sets with other items, like soldiers and military trucks; farm and/or zoo animals. They can also be found where miniature or lighted houses are sold, like the Snow Village® or The Dickens Village®. One can find wooden fences, simulated stone fences, ornate wrought-iron fences, and so on. Real brambles, thorns and all, also make great fences and barriers. Remember, different types of fencing relays something for your client: a white picket fence, or a stone fence built two thick and two high.
- *Gates*—Simple picket fences, ornate wrought iron, arches, oriental gates (such as the *Toriis*—a sacred Japanese gate).
- *Barricades*—Construction barricades, military barricades, traffic barricades.
- *Signs*—Traffic signs (stop, yield, directional, school crossing, traffic cones, etc.), airport signs, street signs.
- *Other*—Railroad tracks.

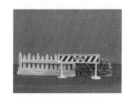

FIGURE 4.6 Fences

Natural Items

- *Sea shells*—Large, small, perfectly complete, broken, pretty, ugly, with barnacles.
- *Vegetation*—Dried seedpods, dried flowers, interestingly shaped branches and twigs, brambles.
- *Rocks*—Colorful, interestingly shaped, fossils, minerals (fool's gold, geodes, quartz, crystals, etc.).

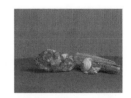

FIGURE 4.7 Natural items

Fantasy

- *Magical*—wizards, witches, cauldrons, wishing well, fairy godmothers, sprites, good witch/bad witch, the Wizard of Oz characters, Lord of the Rings characters.
- *Magical animals*—Dragons, unicorns, Pegasus (winged horse), Centaur, gargoyle, sphinx.
- *Monsters*—Frankenstein, Medusa, werewolf, cyclops, vampire, two-headed beasts, half-human/half-animal.
- *Folklore*—Snow White, Santa Claus/Father Christmas, mermaid.

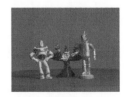

FIGURE 4.8 Fantasy

- *Cartoon and comic book figures*—Figures from some of the classic Disney® cartoons (Mickey & Minnie Mouse, Goofy, Donald Duck), Shrek, Bart Simpson, Betty Boop.
- *Movie characters*—Primary characters from the Wizard of Oz, Inside Out, Cinderella, and even more recent or contemporary animated movies such as Disney's Aladdin, The Little Mermaid, Pocahontas, Frozen, and Star Wars figures. Select other items as well as characters, for example, a flying carpet from Aladdin, ruby-red slippers from the Wizard of Oz, etc. Some of these can be found in the children's meals at fast-food restaurants. Some eateries will let you buy the toy-of-the-week if you choose not to eat the children's meal.
- *Other*—Ghosts, phantoms, gnomes, dwarfs, giants, skeletons.

Spiritual/Mystical

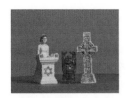

FIGURE 4.9 Spiritual-mystical

- *Religious groups*—Pastors, priests, rabbis, iman/mullah, cross/crucifix, Star of David, crèches/nativity scenes, angels, Bibles, Torah.
- *Other religious groups*—Buddha, Day of the Dead skeletons, Confucius.
- *Mystical*—Magic or crystal balls, crystals, gold, mirrors, chalice, pyramid, gargoyles, Olympians.
- *Other*—Venus, Nile River Goddess, Kali, Shiva, Krishna, Isis.

Landscaping and Other Accessories

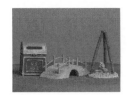

FIGURE 4.10 Landscaping

- *Sky, celestial*—Sun, moon, stars, clouds, rain, rainbow, globe. A pottery sun with a face picked up at a Hispanic market in San Antonio has proven to be a favorite. As soon as it was added to the set, it seemed like every client used it! We have seen other celestial shapes affixed atop a 6- to 8-inch plastic stick that gives the allusion of being the in the "sky" of the sandtray scene.
- *Topographical*—Caves, tunnels, mountains, lakes, volcanoes, fire (sets of flames, campfires, cooking fires). Miniature railroading shops are great sources for these, as are handmade ones from clay and pottery. Clients often make "lakes" by placing small round/oval mirrors in the sand; also by nestling a small container into the sand and filling it with water.
- *Monuments*—Statue of Liberty, Eiffel Tower, Great Pyramids and Great Sphinx, Big Ben, *Arch de Triomphe*, Taj Mahal, Stonehenge, and ones specific to your clientele or area.
- *Other*—Wishing well, treasure chest, treasure ("jewels," gold coins, pearls, glass blobs, marbles), coffin, tombstones, bridge, flags, cannons, snowmen.

Household Items

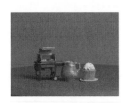

FIGURE 4.11 Household

- *Furniture*—Furniture typical of specific rooms: bedroom, bathroom, living room, kitchen, television set, rocking chair, baby carriage.
- *Tools*—Ladders, wheelbarrow, spades, forks, rakes.
- *Other*—Dishes, utensils, beer and wine bottles, food, garbage cans, party items (decorated cakes, balloons, gift boxes), food, fruit, eating utensils, mailbox, pails, telephones, windmill, benches.

Miscellaneous Items

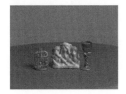

FIGURE 4.12 Other

- *Medical items*—For clients who have experienced some type of chronic illness or medical crisis, these can be very important. Playmobile® makes a nice miniature operating room scene that we have used. We have also used regular-sized syringes (without needles) and even actual pill capsules (it is important to remove the medication and replace with an inert substance such as sugar, in case the client impulsively pops it into his mouth!).

- *Drug/alcohol* —These can be important for persons who have grown up or are currently living in addictive situations. Most hobby stores have miniature wine bottles and beer cans. We know of a colleague who uses the small liquor bottles that can be purchased on airplanes. Also, plastic marijuana leaves, bong, cigarettes, etc.
- *Spatula/brush*—Some clients do not want to touch the sand with their fingers, and need tools to move the sand around. Others enjoy using tools as a means to increase their expression of artistic creation. It is helpful to have a few tools for this purpose.

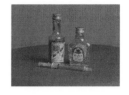

FIGURE 4.13 Addictions

ARRANGEMENT OF MINIATURE FIGURES

The storage and display of the miniature figures are both important issues. There are many options which depend on the space available, how that space is used, and the ways in which you plan to use the sand tray. The method of storage may or may not be the way in which the miniatures are presented to the client. Several examples will be given below.

Regardless of the storage or presentation arrangement, the miniatures should be organized by categories. The categories should always be in the same place. If you are using shelves, a category of items should always be on the same section of the same shelf from one session to another. Or, if the miniatures are in boxes or baskets, these should be placed so that the same category of items is in the same place each time.

There are several reasons for this. The primary one is the ongoing therapeutic need for consistency. Consistency promotes predictability, which promotes safety. Having the categories in the same place allows the clients to locate, from one session to another, the items they wish to select to use. Consistency in the counseling room is particularly important for those clients who have a great deal of chaos in their lives. A related reason for categorizing is for the benefit of clients in a tenuous psychological place. For example, sandtray therapy clients who might want to use a small bunny—if it sits at the feet of an imposing dinosaur, it may be challenging for the emotionally fragile client to reach for it.

Also, consistent arrangement by categories allows the counselor to arrange categories in a sequence that is consistent with the counselor's philosophical view of the client's interaction with the miniatures. For example, we believe that the miniatures should be arranged by primary thematic use. Therefore, the miniatures are placed on thematic continuums. Spiritual and mystical items are placed on the top shelf. On that shelf we would place the positive or "good" first, on the left, then more neutral items in the center, and have the "evil" or negative items last or on the right.

People are on the next shelf. Again, we place across the shelf according to how the items are typically used. The more powerful or aggressive people would be on the far right, such as doctors, rescue personnel, policemen, firemen. If a hobby is hunting, it would go on the right. Gardening, on the other hand is neutral, and would be near the center.

Household items would come next. We see this as a logical sequence, people, and then what they might use. Depending on the size of the shelf, all of these items may be on one shelf, from the dollhouse furniture to the miscellaneous items. Most of these items are neutral and thus could go anywhere. We'd place the beer and wine bottles to the right.

Buildings might be next. Homes on the left, jails and forts on the right, other structures placed in between. Then, vegetation. If there are enough trees of various types, arrange by seasons, spring to winter. Next are the landscaping and other accessories, then the placement of natural items. Animals would follow. This is often the category with the most items. Place domestic or tame animals on the left, with the aggressive on the right, such as lions, tigers, and dinosaurs. All the others, like nonaggressive zoo animals, go in the middle; then fences and signs; then vehicles, fantasy, cartoon, and movies. We think by now you have the idea. We find that some clients want all the powerful, aggressive items for use at first. Other clients only want safe, neutral items initially. This continuum format allows the client to easily find the items desired. Certainly this varies given your number of items and space available.

If you are in a culture that reads right to left, this might be reversed: Our eyes tend to scan visually in the same pattern as we read. Food for thought.

Another benefit of this categorization: it creates an opportunity for the sandtray therapist to see if she has too many or too few items in any of the categories.

If the miniature figures are stored between uses, the consistent placement also speeds up the setup time and cleanup time. The counselor does not have to sort and re-sort the items. It's amazing how quickly one can do so.

OPEN-SHELF ARRANGEMENT

We believe the open-shelf arrangement is optimum (see Figure 4.14). This arrangement allows all of the miniature figures to be openly displayed and the client can easily view what is available. Also, a wall full of toy-like items can put a child at ease. It clearly communicates, "This is a place for kids." Adults often react with curiosity and are attracted to the items, many of which quickly become symbolic of the client's current

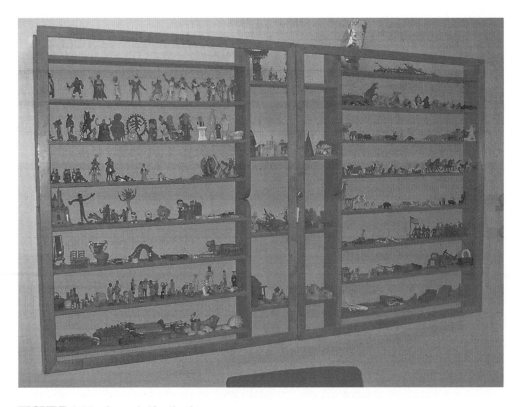

FIGURE 4.14   Open-shelf collection

situation or evoke memories of childhood. The miniature figures also communicate a sense of energy, creativity, and spontaneity. DeDomenico (1995) shares,

> I suspect that the open display evokes a stirring of creative and out world–directed energies innately present in each person. A beautifully tended sandtray display is a statement by the therapist that each person's creative and self-healing energies are welcomed and honored in this place of healing. (p. 73)

Another reason for an open-shelf display is the emotionally fragile client. This client is less likely to rummage through a drawer or a basket of items. We firmly believe that the media, or arrangement thereof, should not be a hindrance to client work.

The open-shelf display does take time to keep neat and clean, with all the miniatures standing, and not just tossed on the shelf. However, we believe it is well worth the time and attention. Shelves inevitably become layered with sand. A can of compressed air held at an angle makes cleaning easy and quick.

An open-shelf display in a setting where several clinicians use the room for a variety of clients and purposes may necessitate some form of doors. Plexiglas doors are effective; the items can still be seen and yet they are safe and secure. Alternatively, wooden doors (or even opaque curtains) may provide for less distraction depending on the needs of others' use of the room, leaving the collection to be easily accessed for a sandtray therapy experience. For clients where a verbal or other form of intervention is planned, the distraction of a miniature collection is thereby avoided. School counselors, for example, often want the miniatures out-of-sight between sessions. We have both used a storage cabinet with doors. With the doors open we have the open-shelf arrangement. However, we have found that the storage cabinet can be dark inside; we have countered this by attaching a light to the door when it is open (an inexpensive clamp-style work light is effective). In fact, we sense that some clients find this underscores the sense of "entering into" a special experience.

A colleague placed 12-inch-deep shelves from floor to ceiling along one end of a room. The shelves are full of a wonderful collection of miniatures. The shelves are white, as are the walls and ceiling. This helps the miniatures stand out visually. A bookcase, also acting as a room divider, holds even more. Two sand trays and a couple of upholstered chairs complete the sandtray therapy space. It's ever so inviting and warm! However, access to the upper shelves can be a challenge, so a step-stool is a help.

Another open-shelf variation we've seen used is a closet attached to the counseling room. All three walls of the closet were lined with narrow shelves from top to bottom. The clients simply move between the closet and the sand tray. The sand tray, on a rolling cart, is stored in the closet between sessions. If available, this is a very nice arrangement for a room that has multiple purposes for several clinicians.

BASKETS OR BOXES

Some counselors do not have the space for an open-shelf arrangement. Therefore, many therapists use baskets or boxes, typically one for each category. Another possibility is using limited shelf space for the more fragile items with the rest of the figures placed in other containers.

The baskets/boxes generally work well, although it is more time consuming for the client to rummage through a basket/box full of animals to see if just what is wanted is there. We hear mixed reports from counselors who use this system. Some indicate that the client freely utilizes the miniatures, even with the need of a bit more time to construct a sandtray. Others believe that the items in the baskets/boxes are not used as much as those on the shelves. When putting out the baskets/boxes for a session, as indicated previously, it is important to consistently arrange them in the same order or placement, so the client can more easily find what is needed.

Whatever the chosen arrangement, it goes back to a philosophical view of the individual clinician using sandtray therapy: What is my belief regarding the client's interaction with miniature figures and the sand tray to provide the optimal therapeutic experience? Lowenfeld (Thompson, 1990, p. 12) preferred a cabinet with drawers based on her belief in the need to control the amount and kind of sensory stimulation. Kalff preferred shelves (Thompson, 1990, p. 13). Thompson controls for the "danger of . . . being overwhelmed" by arranging the room so the shelves are at the client's back while building in the tray (1990, p. 13). The reader's decision might result in a combination of open shelves and drawers, boxes, baskets, or other containers. Or, it might be by limiting the overall number of miniature figures in the collection. Whatever one chooses, it should be the result of an intentional, thoughtful, informed decision (Homeyer & Sweeney, in press).

PORTABLE SET USING BOXES

For some individuals, a portable set of miniature figures is needed. Some school counselors move from school to school, some counselors provide in-home therapy; students in university practicum clinics may need the flexibility to use the sand tray in any of the clinic rooms. We have found the use of tackle boxes (as in fishing tackle) to be quite adequate. Available in a variety of sizes, one or more categories can be placed in a tackle box. The tackle boxes have flexibility, having movable vertical partitions to allow for the making of larger or smaller compartments (see Figure 4.15).

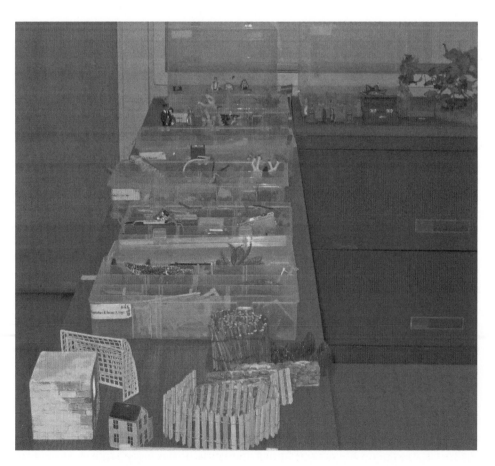

FIGURE 4.15   Box collection

When set out for a session, categories can easily be arranged in a standard manner. The lids easily pop off for ease of setting up in a small space. It works well to stand up some of the miniatures, placing some outside the box on the table or floor. This allows for easier viewing by the client. We believe that a pleasing, eye appealing presentation is important: It communicates to the clients that this place is prepared for them and their anticipated work is respected and honored.

A portable sand tray kit is easily put into a wheeled suitcase, which can be taken in an automobile or on an airplane. The boxes also sit well on a shelf of a wheeled cart, with the sand tray on top, for easy moving around a building or a clinic. When the boxes are closed they are neatly secure.

SOURCES OF MINIATURE FIGURES

As indicated earlier, after a while we can find miniature figures wherever we seem to go! But initial sources, which are often overlooked, are friends who may have toys no longer being used by their children, garage sales, and rummage sales. If you are working in a school, let teachers and staff know what you are looking for and ask for donations to the set. Other sources are

- Craft and hobby shops
- Souvenir and novelty shops
- Model railroad stores
- Cake decorating suppliers
- Toy stores
- Nature centers
- Gift shops
- Aquarium supply stores
- Vendors at play therapy and sandplay conferences

Some specific vendors who specialize in both the common and more unusual or hard-to-find miniatures are listed in Appendix B.

AN INITIAL SET

Putting together an initial or basic set of miniatures can seem like a daunting and expensive task. However, we recommend to the person gathering together the first set of miniatures to develop a basic, but broad, collection. Then, continue to add to it as one can. Here are some hints for an easy and quick beginning.

- Sets of toys: Some toy stores will carry complete sets that will give you a variety of items for several categories. For example, a vehicle set was recently purchased that had 45 items. It included many different types of cars and trucks, two helicopters, a motorcycle, barricades, street signs, traffic cones, firemen, and policemen. Purchased at a toy store at an outlet mall it was very inexpensive. The same experience has been found with farm sets (animals, fences, a barn, farm workers, tractor and wagon, and trees). Same for a zoo set (lots of animals, including flamingos, fences, cages [often used as a jail], zoo workers, trees, plants, pond, and a building). Clearly, this is a great way to begin the collection of several categories!
- Bags of toys: Small bags of soldiers often include a tank, jeep, and military airplane. Bags of cowboys and Indians often have horses, a teepee, a totem pole, a canoe, and a covered wagon. A third collection of items that is frequently found

includes astronauts, a rocket, a shuttle, and a U.S. flag. These bags include, obviously, items from several categories, in addition to a variety and initially adequate number of people (only needing to add more babies and families). A shopping trip resulted in a package of bugs, small snakes, frogs, and lizards, five of each, for a few dollars each. Sacks of dinosaurs, horses, zoo animals, dolphins, fishes, etc. are easily found. And a small sack usually provides enough items for a beginning set. Bags like these are typically found in the toy section of grocery stores, as well as toy stores, of course. The bags are usually only a few dollars each. The items below are also often found in similar places.

■ Bridges are very important! The aquarium section of a store is the easiest place to locate one. More elaborate (and more expensive) bridges can be located at model railroading stores. Model railroad stores are also great for a wide variety of landscaping items: trees, rocks, caves, tunnels, etc. Houses and a variety of buildings are also readily available.

To obtain some of the more unique items, go to the cake decorating section of a party store or arts and crafts store. These are areas to find items such as the following:

■ Babies, highchairs, strollers
■ Brides, grooms, attendants
■ Graduates, Bar/Bat Mitzvah figures
■ Miniature bouquet of balloons, gift boxes
■ Wine and alcohol bottles

Seasonal decorating items make the following easy to obtain:

■ Halloween: witches, ghosts, cauldrons, tombstones, coffins.
■ Christmas: angels, nativity sets (which can be quite elaborate and extensive to include, camels, sheep, campfires, small structures, angels, Mary and child, Joseph, shepherds, Wise Men, etc.).
■ Also at Christmas it is easy to find small houses, trees, and a variety of fences (picket fences, stone fences, wrought iron fences, etc.). This is where you will find quite a variety of fences with gates. Gates can otherwise be difficult to locate.
■ Hanukkah provides menorahs, dreidels, and Stars of David.

Also give thought to your local clinical and geographic populations. Think of the clients you will be serving in your unique setting.

■ University? A few graduates figures, miniature books, alcohol bottles, etc.
■ Active or retired military? Additional military figures (including finding a few that are unique, like generals, etc., to supplement the typical 'army-men'; more tents, vehicles).
■ Adolescents? Drug bottles, syringes, cars, graduate figures.
■ Middle school? Horses for the girls; creepy-crawlies of all kinds for the boys.
■ Hospice/Elderly? Additional spiritual items, bridges (crossing-over), tomb stones.

You get the idea. So give some thought to this for your initial set, so that you will not only have a wide variety of tangible words and symbols, but those specific to the clinical population you serve.

Basic Sandtray Miniature Set Shopping List
(Approximately 300 items)

□ People
__ families, two or more
__ babies, four (different poses, if possible)
__ bride and groom
__ occupational (police, firemen, construction
     workers, etc.)
__ army, 16 or so
__ astronauts or knights

□ Animals
__ dinosaurs, four
__ zoo: lions, giraffes, zebra, elephants, six to eight
__ domestic: cows, horses, sheep, six to eight
     (if working with preteens, six to eight horses)
__ insects, spiders, snakes
__ sea animals

□ Vegetation
__ trees, four to six
__ plants, flowers

□ Buildings
__ houses, two
__ school (especially if working with children)
__ lighthouse
__ castle, fort, or teepee
__ jail

□ Vehicles
__ cars, four
__ trucks, two
__ airplane, one
__ boat, one
__ helicopter, one
__ police car, ambulance, other rescue vehicle

□ Fences and signs
__ fences, about 36 inches
__ traffic signs, three to four
__ barricades, three to four

□ Natural items
__ sea shells, six to ten
__ vegetation, twigs

__ rocks, five to six, plain and polished
__ Fool's gold
__ crystals

□ Fantasy
__ wizard
__ fairy godmother
__ dragons, two
__ monsters, four to six
__ cartoon figures, four
__ space aliens, two to four

□ Spiritual / mystical
__ angels
__ Cross
__ Buddha
__ Madonna
__ Star of David, menorah
__ small mirrors

□ Landscaping and other accessories
__ wishing well
__ bridges, two to three
__ treasure chest
__ treasure, gold coins
__ cannon
__ flags, four of various types

□ Household items
__ furniture
__ tools
__ garbage can
__ mailbox
__ windmill
__ food

□ Client-specific items (make your own list; see
     section above)

— _____
— _____
— _____
— _____

5

Protocol for a Sandtray Therapy Session

Sandtray therapy is used in individual sessions, joint/dyad, or group/family sessions; anytime there is one or more person(s) in the room. The use of the sand tray, as with any therapeutic intervention or technique, should be purposeful, intentional, and selected for a specific goal. Before conducting a sandtray therapy session you should be clear regarding the purpose for using the sand tray with this particular client at this particular time in the overall intervention process.

CLIENT ISSUES TO CONSIDER

For What Age Client Is Sandtray Therapy Appropriate?

A wide age range of clients can benefit from work in the sand tray. Developmental considerations must be taken into account and its impact on the use of the materials.

- Young children, 3–6 years of age, can be expected to use the miniature figures and sand tray as an active, dynamic play experience. It may, in fact, look more like play therapy in miniature. In such instances, the counselor may do verbal tracking as one might do in a more traditional play therapy setting. The dynamic play of this age group is also why some counselors prefer to use traditional play therapy rather than sandtray therapy with young children.
- Older children are able to sufficiently delay the impulse to play in order to create a scene in the sand tray (unless seriously regressed in play because of experienced trauma). However, some older children will continue to play with or transform the initial scene during or after the discussion of the scene in the tray.
- Adolescents are often attracted to sand tray because of the optional nonverbal use. Adolescents often have a difficult time talking about feelings and expressing what is troubling them. Sandtray therapy can provide a nonverbal mode of communication which engages adolescents and may lead to verbal interactions. A note on doing sandtray therapy with adolescents: Many teens are acutely aware of therapists who do play therapy with children. Not wanting to appear immature, their response to the suggestion of 'working/playing in the sand' may well be, "I don't want any part of that play therapy stuff—that's for little kids." We have found that a response to adolescent reluctance can be something like: "Of course I wouldn't do play therapy with you. You're a whole lot closer to being an adult than being a kid. I wouldn't insult you by asking you to do play therapy. However, there is another kind of counseling that I do with adults. It's called sandtray counseling/therapy, and I'm thinking you're mature enough for it." It may seem like we're giving them a line, but it is a true statement, and we've found it engages teens almost every time. The counselor's own resonance of

authenticity and belief that a sandtray experience would be helpful for the teen client is imperative in engaging the teen, and any age client, for that matter.

■ Adults of all ages are able to use the sand tray materials successfully. Adults may occasionally be resistant (much like adolescents), thinking that sand tray work is too juvenile in which to engage. Our experience is this concern arises more often in couples and family therapy than in sessions with individuals because the adult is concerned about the other's reactions. The sandtray therapy experience actually creates a valuable opportunity to engage partners and adult family members in the counseling process: "I know it may seem a little strange, or even childish. But I also know that you're invested in seeing things change—simply by the fact that you've taken the time to come in here. I can also see how much you care about your partner/family member. I'm wondering if you can translate that investment—that care—into trying this different way of doing a session." This may give the impression we're suggesting manipulating people to participate; this isn't the intent, but rather it speaks directly to their desire for change. And it works!

WHEN IS A GOOD TIME TO USE SANDTRAY THERAPY?

Some therapists use sandtray therapy as the sole or primary intervention with clients. While this may be the appropriate choice for some therapists or clients, we suggest that there are times in the therapeutic process that may particularly prove amenable to sandtray intervention. These are generic suggestions acknowledging the therapeutic intent is always considered.

■ As an introduction to counseling. This is especially true for clients who are reluctant or resistive to the counseling process. This is a uniquely different and unexpected experience and way to develop the therapeutic alliance.

■ As a change of pace. Clients who have been in talk therapy for some length of time may be reenergized or able to refocus. Adolescents, like those in foster care, may have experienced years of counseling. Sandtray work can offer a much needed change. It may also serve as a method to express feelings and issues that are difficult to access with typical talk therapy.

■ An opportunity to evaluate the progress in therapy. Viewing a sequence of the pictures of client sandtrays can reveal progress over time and allow for assessment of change. This can additionally validate the clinician's assessment of the primary mode of intervention. Also, we use a sandtray therapy session periodically with an older child with whom we are doing traditional play therapy. The periodic work in the tray provides an additional way to assess the child's progress. Also, we may have a caregiver-child sandtray session to evaluate improvement in their relationship or improvement of parenting issues.

WHAT TYPE OF CLIENT BENEFITS FROM SANDTRAY THERAPY?

Although we touched upon this in the discussion of rationale in Chapter 2, it is important to revisit those client populations who may especially benefit from the therapeutic modality of sandtray. Weinrib (1983) suggests several categories:

■ For those clients who are introverted and tense. The tactile interaction with the sand reduces tension and anxiety. Clients may simply move their hands through the sand or let the sand stream through their fingers. We've experienced many teenagers and young adults who are able to talk more freely when one hand is moving through the sand. This resulting experience of the client's ability to self-regulate, calming parts of the brain, benefits the client in two ways: the ability to begin to verbally interact in session and experiencing the ability to manage anxiety. Handling the miniature figures can also provide a positive tactile experience. The texture of items, more often those made of natural materials, neurologically serves as a way for clients to reconnect with their feelings (more on this in Chapter 10).

■ For those clients who are hyperactive and/or have hysterical tendencies. Creating a scene in the sand tray can assist clients to focus. Selecting miniature figures and placing them in the sand tray provides the space for clients to externalize and objectify their issues. As with some art techniques, the focus of discussion can then become what has been created in the tray, 'containing' both clients and their work. Soothing tactile interaction with the media may also reduce the frenetic aspects of their behavior. Ryce-Menuhin (1992) discusses the use of sandtray therapy with the adult "hysteric". He indicates that the holding quality of the sand tray has a positive impact on the hysteric's boundary issues. He recommends providing "intensive short periods of sandplay followed by a cessation of 3 months, then again an intensive series of sandplays" (p. 35). The time period between the intensive sandtray experiences allows the adult hysteric the time needed to gradually reduce the unbounded, acting-out behavior. The opportunity to move physically around the tray, back-and-forth between the tray and the miniature figure collection, is beneficial. Also useful is the opportunity to expand their work beyond the tray to the table on which the tray may sit or onto the rim of the sand tray (if these are available).

■ For those clients who over-verbalize. Some clients over-verbalize as a defense mechanism, or an avoidance or resistance measure. The optional nonverbal experience provides a different methodology and thereby bypasses these forms of interference of the therapeutic process. Sometimes clients over-verbalize because they do not know how to get to their real issues or feelings. Sandtray therapy can promote access to these core concerns. The client does not need to find the "right words" because the communication occurs without words, via the scene in the tray.

  □ Additionally, similar to art therapy, the externalizing of a client's issues in a concrete form gives the therapeutic issue form and substance. This may not otherwise occur for some clients. Confined within the parameters of the sand tray the client may develop the ability to be likewise appropriately restrained. The sides of the sand tray physically provide the containment of and boundaries around the client's scene, assisting the client to likewise internalize needed boundaries. Miniature figures of containers (cups, pots, boxes, baskets, and such) used within the tray are also available for these purposes.

■ For those clients who rationalize and/or intellectualize. Rationalization and intellectualization serve essentially the same purpose as over-verbalization: resistance to the therapeutic process. Often these are defense mechanisms that the client has used for so long that it seems impossible (for both the client and therapist) to move beyond them. Similar to the client who over-verbalizes, work in the sand tray facilitates moving past the resistance.

☐ Additionally, clients who rationalize and/or intellectualize often have difficulty getting in touch with their feelings. Sandtray therapy is noted for its ability to bring to awareness the emotional aspects of a client's issues. As such, it should be used wisely and with an understanding of the possible impact. Some clients, discussing their creation in the tray, discover more has been disclosed than intended, especially at a feeling level. For clients who are not comfortable with their own feelings, this can be a distressing realization. Edith Kramer (1972), the child art therapist, wrote that children 'betray' themselves in their artwork. Similarly, people of all ages may also 'voice' more about themselves in their sandtray than they expected or intended. It is crucial that the counselor using sandtray is aware of this possibility.

■ For those clients who have trouble verbalizing. Clearly, a nonverbal experience is an asset for clients who have difficulty talking. This challenge may include clients with speech difficulties or who are ashamed of their limited vocabulary or speaking ability. The sandtray can be a wonderfully freeing experience for this type of client. Depending on the perspective and intentionality of the counselor, the client who has difficulty verbalizing may be given the opportunity to work in the sandtray without any follow-up verbal processing or discussion. Some sandtray therapists have clients journal about their sandtray work between sessions. This may include their narrative about the created scene and their self-awareness during the building process. Journaling is used in a sandtray therapy class with graduate students (both when working as the client and as the sandtray therapist). The resulting insight is extremely valuable and expands the educational and experiential experience.

☐ School counselors report positive change in students when provided an opportunity to work non-verbally in the sand and then given the choice of whether to talk about it afterward. Reportedly, many who choose not to talk about their work in the sand benefit from it. Wheat (1995) reports the use of a sand tray by classroom teachers. Each student is scheduled a regular time to work in the sand tray each week. The teachers occasionally observe the process but no verbal interaction occurs between the teacher and student. One teacher reported, "I also find this form of quiet and meditative self-expression balances out the other 'louder' activities happening in the room" (p. 83). Wheat also states "implementing therapeutic sand play is one important step in helping children deal with their emotions and thereby attain inner peace" (p. 83).

PROTOCOL FOR CONDUCTING A SESSION

Six-Step Protocol

1. Room preparation
2. Introduction to the client
3. Creation in the sandtray
4. Post-creation
5. Sand tray cleanup
6. Documenting the session

How the sandtray session is conducted is influenced by the sandtray therapist's approach or theory. We suggest therapists, within their current working model, take the time to develop the steps to their own sandtray therapy sessions, thoughtfully and intentionally, prior to implementation and working with clients. We offer here a general protocol to conduct a sandtray therapy session, recommending six key steps. These are helpful for a review of possible components to anyone integrating sandtray therapy to the way in which one is already working with clients. Our protocol is easily adapted for most counseling theories through the prompts given to the client and the way in which the created tray is processed (more of that in Chapters 6 and 7).

Step One: Room Preparation

This process will vary depending on your particular situation. As indicated in the previous chapter, some clinicians may have a separate sandtray therapy space. In this case, the pre-session preparation is simple:

■ Review the room to be sure the sandtray(s) and miniature figures are in place.

■ Check to be sure that the sand tray has no buried items from a previous session, which can be easily overlooked. This is especially important if you share the room and materials.

■ The sand should be level and mostly smooth, providing your client with a neutral point from which to begin.

If you use two sand trays:

■ Check the wet tray for sufficient moisture in the sand. Or, if you allow the client to add the water, be sure the water container is full. Again, if you share a sand tray room this will be particularly necessary.

If you use one sand tray:

■ Be sure there is a minimal, but sufficient, amount of water. Some therapists provide a limited amount of water in a spray bottle. Providing this, or some other small container, is appropriate. This reduces the possibility of the client intentionally or accidentally over-wetting the sand. This is important if you, or a colleague, must use the sand tray throughout the same day.

Left uncovered, most slightly wet sand will dry sufficiently overnight. This is not the case where a substantial amount of water has been used. To help dry overly-wet sand, at the end of the day, mound-up the sand like a mountain or volcano. This provides increased surface area for drying. Increasing air flow with a small fan also helps for extremely soggy sand. Remember it can be very dismaying for a client to come in to a tray full of very wet or soupy sand. It will directly impact that client's work in the sand.

If you work in a multipurpose room, where you have to set-out the figures for sessions, remember to arrange the miniature figures by categories in a consistent manner (see Chapter 4). This allows the client to access the items from a consistent, non-chaotic arrangement. Our experience has been that putting out the boxes of miniature figures becomes a quick and easy task, especially if they are returned to the appropriate storage spot after each use.

Place the therapists' chair in a nonintrusive place, slightly removed from the sand tray and miniature collection, but still close enough for easy viewing of the client working in the sand. The client should be able to sense that the therapist is fully observant of the creative process in the sand tray, but not intrusive in the developing dynamic between the client and the media. Arrange the other furniture in the room to facilitate client movement between the sandtray(s) and the collection of miniature figures. There should be a clear path between the tray and miniatures. It is counterproductive for the client to get frustrated if there are tables, chairs, or other items to navigate around each time the selection of another figure is desired. It is helpful if the client is able to walk completely around the tray, which facilitates greater access to the entire tray from several perspectives.

Also, depending on your miniature display, you may need to provide a step stool of some type to help the client access items placed on high shelves. This does carry a liability concern, so be careful! Placement of shelves is a consideration during the initial setting up the sandtray therapy room. Shelves might be placed on the floor for children; attached to a wall, higher or lower, depending on use by children or adults.

Step Two: Introduce the Sand Tray and Miniature Figures

The initial introduction of the experience to the client may include the therapist walking to the sand tray, moving the sand with her hand, demonstrating the blue bottom, and the location of water for possible use. Then, 'introduce' the miniature figures, mentioning some of the primary categories. Perhaps also indicate that the client can use as many or few as wanted and also the use of a small basket to gather the figures to take them to the sand tray. The prompt or instruction to the client will be based on the purpose for which you are using this technique. The prompt may be directive or nondirective in nature, or both. It is important to have this thought through before the beginning of the session, so your prompt can be clearly and concisely worded.

Nondirective

You may choose to give minimal or no specific directions at all to the client. This allows the scene in the sand to be a result of the client's interaction with the miniatures and the sand. This can be a very exciting, powerful, and meaningful experience. In this case, the counselor might introduce the experience something like this: "I would like you to take a few moments to look at the figures, and then select a few that really 'speak to you.' Place them in the sand (point to the sand tray). Then add as many as you like to create a world in the sand. I will sit here quietly until you are finished. Take your time and let me know when you are done."

With older children and teenagers, one might use the following prompt: "I'd like you to build a scene in the sand. It can be a scene of anything you want." If the child or teenager looks confused or unsure of what is expected, it is possible to continue by saying, "You know how if you are watching a movie you can push the 'pause' button? The movie stops and you can see only one scene of the movie. This scene in the sand could be like that, not from a movie, but anything you can think up on your own. Just look over the miniatures and put in the sand the ones you like and go from there." Generally, this is enough to help the client get started. Some clients will begin before the prompt is completed.

Some clinicians prefer using particular words, such as

- create a world,
- create your world,
- create a scene,
- build a world,
- build your world, or
- build a scene

when introducing the experience. Use whatever works for you and with which you feel most comfortable. The words used to provide instructions to the client can impact in various ways.

Directive

Other clients may be overwhelmed with such an unstructured experience. In these cases, giving a specific task may be more productive. Also, the therapist might want to tie the experience to the client's ongoing therapeutic issue(s). For example, with a college-age client who is having roommate problems, we might give the following prompt: "Make a scene in the sand that expresses how you feel when you come home after class to find that your roommates have broken the house rules again."

Step Three: The Client Creates the Scene in the Sand Tray

Allow the client time to complete the building of a scene in the sand tray. Meanwhile, the therapist honors both the process that is occurring (the building or creating) and the product (scene) that is being formed.

Counselor's Role

Counselors speak of the importance of 'containing' or 'holding' within all counseling sessions; Jungians label it the 'free and protected space'. Regardless of theoretical orientation, this is an important enough concept to discuss as it relates specifically to sandtray therapy. Developing, maintaining, and containing the therapeutic environment in which the client does his or her work (verbal or nonverbal) is crucial in any form of psychotherapy. This 'holding environment' or 'free and protected space' is a must and is the responsibility of the counselor. This involves the concept of *temenos* discussed earlier—the therapy and the sand tray itself providing a boundary between the sacred and the profane. The client must believe (know, think, feel) he or she is safe—emotionally, psychologically, spiritually, and physically.

> In an emotional sense the therapist "enters" the sandtray with the patient and participates empathically in the act of creation (Weinrib, 1983, p. 30).

Critical is the ability of the therapist to assimilate the feeling and atmosphere of the process and the individual scenes in the sand. In an emotional sense the therapist "enters" the sandtray with the client and participates empathetically, attuned to the act of creation, thus establishing a profound and wordless rapport. The silent capacity to enter into the creation of his world with the client can, in itself, help repair the feeling of isolation with which so many clients are afflicted (Weinrib, 1983, p. 30).

Therefore, while the client is building and creating in the tray, the counselor must be fully present. One must listen, observe, and participate empathically and cognitively, thus sharing in the act of creation. There should be resonating and attunement which we now know is neurobiologically based (Badenoch, 2008). It's admittedly hard work to be fully present without talking, especially for those clinicians who have been verbally dependent in therapeutic relationships. Some of you who are reading this, and have not experienced the more nonverbal processes (sandtray therapy, play therapy, art therapy, expressive arts, etc.), may find that not talking is a new, and perhaps difficult, experience. *Trust the process.* This is crucial. To learn to be attuned and fully present, with the willingness to resonate with the client, while maintaining the free and protected space, observing the client's process while building and creating the product may take a bit of time and practice. But it's mandatory!

Of course, as soon as we suggest keeping verbalization to a minimum, we also begin thinking of exceptions. A primary exception would be using sand tray with young children. As stated above, with young children the sand tray process may well be similar to doing play therapy in miniature. It would be appropriate for the counselor to track the child's play as in play therapy. Young children are more apt to use the miniatures as toys (which they are) and develop sequences of active, dynamic play full of movement and sounds as in a typical play therapy session. We believe this is fine. This takes into consideration the child's developmental level thereby modifying the sandtray approach appropriately (read more of this in Chapter 11).

Other exceptions to the admonition to be silent while the client is creating in the sand are tied to the therapeutic purpose. If the purpose is to help the reticent, withdrawn client loosen up and relax, and this happily results with the client beginning to talk, then we would support that client by dialoguing. If, however, the counselor chose a sandtray therapy experience to help the over-verbalizing client to focus, then we might respond to that client who is attempting to engage the therapist in a discussion while creating a tray, with something like: "I would like you to finish the sandtray, and then we'll talk." Brief, and to the point; inherently discouraging a response. Again, it is imperative that the counselor is aware of the intention and purpose for using sandtray therapy with the client. This will assist the counselor in knowing the appropriate responses.

The Process and the Product

Understanding the Process

- *Ease/difficult*
- *Determined/hesitant*
- *Able/unable to be fully involved*
- *Purposeful/nonpurposeful*
- *Plans ahead/constructs as it happens*

The product (the completed tray) is obviously important and where many novice sandtray therapists focus their time and energy. At the same time, observing the client's process while building in the tray is equally important. In traditional talk therapy, counselors are trained to pay attention to nonverbal communication by the client. This continues to be informative in sandtray work, except that in addition, attention is paid to the client's approach and carry-through of the task of building the scene in the sand tray.

Understanding the process includes dynamics such as the following questions: Does the client appear to find building as an easy or difficult task? Is the client determined or hesitant in selection of the figures and construction in the tray? Is the client able or unable to be fully involved in the entire creation experience? Does the work appear purposeful or non-purposeful (random)? Does the client begin with a plan, or does the construction in the tray seem to be created as the building happens? Understanding the client and how his or her particular issues begin to be expressed in the client's approach to the process may also provide the clinician with other dynamics for which to watch.

An additional area of observation during the process of building the sandtray is how the client interacts with the media. First, the sand: Does the client spend a great deal of time smoothing and re-smoothing the surface? Is the sand moved about, piled up here, exposing the blue bottom of the box there? In damp sand, are tunnels made? Or complete opposite, does the client carefully make sure not to touch the sand at all? Second, the client's interaction with the miniature figures: Does the client avoid certain objects or complete categories? Linger over others? Carefully, even reverently, handle others? Stroking, touching, and caressing particular miniatures? Does the client begin with an apparent focus and plan, but a shift occurs that leaves the tray in chaos?

Many counselors feel comfortable subtly taking a few notes during the session. The notes can be referred to during the discussion or processing time, which may come next. Others believe any note taking influences the client. We suggest the sandtray therapist be thoughtful regarding the use of notetaking.

Step Four: The Post-Creation Phase

Once again, your purpose for having your client create or build a scene in the sand will impact this step. Some counselors prefer to allow the creative process, which activates the client's internal healing process, to stand on its own. These clinicians will not discuss or verbally process the creation in the sand tray.

Others will use the scene in the sand tray as a springboard for discussion and continued verbal work with the client. Some will have clients move figures within the tray, or add/remove figures as the discussion continues. There are many therapeutic uses of the scene created in the sand. Clients discover insights for themselves regardless of whether it is a directed or nondirected experience. Counselors can be very tempted to interpret the symbolism of the miniatures and the meaning of a scene for the client. Resist! While the counselor may have insight into typical meanings, or thoughts about the significance for a particular client, it is the meaning attributed by the client that is the most important. It is the counselor's skillful asking of questions and assisting the client in the exploration of the communication within the sandtray scene that is the real challenge for the counselor.

Discussing or Processing the Sandtray Scene

We will provide a more detailed discussion of this process in the following chapter. Knowing, however, some of the classic or typical interpretations of the sandtray scene and/or miniature figures may provide the counselor with some insight or guidance as the sandtray therapy session moves into the phase of processing of the created scene.

Visually Observe the Completed Sandtray

Although the counselor has been observing the continuing development of the scene in the sandtray, it is important to stop and take a moment to view the completed sandtray in its entirety. As previously noted, one reason for the dimensions of the classic sand tray is that the entire scene can be visually perceived as a single unit. This also communicates to the clients the value you place on their world. It honors and respects them. It also provides some time for the client to mentally and emotionally shift from the creating mode to the processing mode.

Emotionally Observe the Sandtray

What is the emotional content? What emotion does the sandtray creation evoke in the counselor? Is it warm, comforting? Peaceful? Angry? Conflicted? Cold? In our experience of supervising counselors, we have noticed that too few counselors, regardless of the treatment approach, check in with or trust their own emotional responses.

A caution needs to be mentioned here. While it is very helpful to monitor and use our own emotional response, we must be equally aware that clients easily pick up on the affective state of the therapist. If you are having a bad day, it will not only affect the way you provide therapy, but clients pick up on your bad mood and introject the assumption that they have done something wrong or are having a bad day as well! Our understanding of attunement and resonance continues to be informed by neurobiological research. We can reap the benefits, or increase client dissonance.

Evaluate the Organization of the Tray

Analytically trained psychotherapists who use sandtray therapy may spend a great deal of time in the assessment or interpretation of the structural organization of the sandtray. We are not attempting to train or inform clinicians reading this manual to use the sand tray in that manner. Our focus rather, is simply in the use of sandtray as a therapeutic technique. Having said this, personal experience has shown certain aspects of the arrangement of the miniature figures and use of the sand within the sand tray to be helpful in working with a given client. The following "classic" organizations of miniature figures in the sand tray are modifications of Charlotte Bühler's research. (We offer a much more detailed discussion of her work in Chapter 11). We have found these possibilities, based in early research, provide the novice sandtray therapist with clinical hunches of client issues. These are seen as a beginning platform from which to begin the discussion of the sandtray creation.

1. **An Empty World**. A sandtray is considered an Empty World if there are less than 50 items used in the tray, and less than five different categories. An empty world may be reflective of the client viewing his/her world as an unhappy, empty place; or that the client feels rejected, desires to escape; or may be unable to be creative because of depressive symptoms. Bühler (1951b) indicated people building Empty Worlds may be emotionally blocking (not too many items in

Understanding the Process

1. Empty Worlds
2. Distorted Worlds
3. Aggressive Worlds

the tray, resulting in a scene without rich detail) or emotionally fixated (using only a few categories).

A sandtray is also considered empty if there are no people in the sandtray. In this case, people are defined as men, women, children, occupational figures, and so on. Bühler (1951b) shared her findings that when adults used only children in their trays, it is a reflection of "exceptional insecurity and regression" (p. 73). Soldiers are not considered to be counted as people. Soldiers are so typically used in play to symbolize aggression that the sandtray client typically uses them as "non-people." There are, however, always those exceptions, such as if your client is part of a military community. An unpeopled world may reflect the client's wish to escape and/or is an expression of hostile feelings toward people. Certainly, children who have been abused may build an unpeopled world because people in their real world have hurt them and the children *do* want to escape their world. Understandably, these children have a great deal of anger and hostility toward those people who have hurt them emotionally, psychologically, spiritually, physically, and/or sexually.

2. **A Distorted World**. A Distorted World has three subtypes of organization: Closed/Fenced, Disorganized, and Rigid. The Closed/Fenced configuration is identified when the client uses fences or other items to divide the scene in the sandtray. This configuration is used so often by clients that it is crucial to have many options of fencing or barrier material from which the client may choose. Highly anxious clients will place fencing or barriers in their trays first, a sign of an unusually high need for protection (Bühler, 1951b). A scene is more correctly identified as Closed if most of the miniature figures and items are *within* the fenced area; it is Fenced if the figures are *outside* the perimeter of the enclosed area. A Closed arrangement is seen as the client expressing one or more of the following through putting the figures within the enclosed area, such as

   ☐ needing to be protective (of self and/or others placed within the fenced area)
   ☐ self-isolating, closing self off from others (managing insecurity)
   ☐ identifying with the figures within the enclosed area
   ☐ confining and imprisoning symbols of danger.

And a Fenced organization, dividing the tray into areas may be the client's

■ fearing his/her own inner impulses (a need for external controls in many areas of the world)
■ needing to compartmentalize (to manage anxiety)
■ closing dangers out.

A Rigid scene is sometimes called a 'World of Rows' or a 'Schematic Arrangement'. The arrangement of the items appears unrealistic, with a rigid arrangement, typically in rows or some clearly geometric pattern. This may be understood as an extreme need for order, as a reaction to the client's chaotic world. It is also possible that the client has a great need for perfectionism or self-control. The client may also be emotionally rigid or repressed. Bühler (1951b) indicates it is the "gravest sign" reflective of obsessive compulsivity. The "deepest anxiety expresses itself within in row arrangements or in chaotic constructions" (Bühler, 1951b, p. 74). A note here, however, is that a circle or square may be a mandala, and is not seen as a rigid geometric shape. A mandala is seen as a form of centering and wholeness and is viewed as a positive sign in the therapeutic process. Understanding the quality and content of the shape is essential.

The third sub-type of the Distorted World is Disorganized, sometimes labeled as incoherent or chaotic. The Distorted arrangement displays items placed in a chaotic, impulsive manner. These trays clearly *look* chaotic and would be noted as such. While watching the process of the building taking place, the client might have begun in a deliberate and planful manner, but then loses the ego control to continue, deteriorating into chaos. A world of this type may indicate that the client is

- showing his/her own inner confusion
- reflecting the chaos of his/her own world
- unable to maintain self-control.

Other indicators of Disorganized would be items in odd placements, a tiger in an otherwise neutral or positive scene, like that of a neighborhood, or a house in the middle of a body of water (unless there had been recent flooding).

3. **An Aggressive World**. Finally, the Aggressive World is also easily identified. It may take the form of a battle scene with soldiers or other characters fighting; car, bus, boat, or airplane crashes; or wild animal attacks (attacking other animals, people, and/or vehicles). Some of the scenes may seem more socially acceptable, for example, scenes of athletic competition; other scenes may be more unacceptable, for example, animals and bugs attacking people, angels, or babies.

The meaning of an Aggressive World is just that—aggression. We should not be surprised by some clients who build aggressive worlds because they may be acting out in some manner in their own world. Others may surprise us, however. This may be the client who is internalizing anger and uses the safety of the sandtray to express his/her anger. There may be a very real reason for these clients to be afraid of acting out in their personal, real environment, such as in the case of domestic violence.

Bühler (1951b) indicates that Aggressive Worlds may be the less severe of all of her findings of the clinical signs in the sand tray. Her research found that the Aggressive Worlds can indicate a "more pronounced aggressiveness" if built in the client's first tray; deeper resentment might be present if there are a number of different accidents within a single tray (p. 72).

Identify the Theme or Metaphor of the Content

If the sandtray scene or world is one of the above, then the theme may be easy to identify. Often, it is not that simple. (Yes, we know, counseling is rarely so simple.)

Sometimes, it may be more communicative to identify the metaphor of the sandtray rather than a specific theme. For example, when a 12-year-old girl expressed the intensity of her first serious crush, she had the fence (which had been carefully surrounding figures for several sessions) lying down, as if blown down from energy that exploded from inside the fenced area. Identifying this scene as "the energy of love" is much more communicative of the content than attempting a thematic label.

Once the clinician has completed the above steps, then the invitation to discuss the scene can occur. An opening question that we particularly like to use is: "What title would you give this scene/world?" John Allan (2007) shared, for example, during a play therapy training event that after a child paints a picture, he invites the child to discuss the painting, first asking for a possible title. Badenoch (2008) suggests using a question regarding the feeling in the tray as a way to move more gently from the right-brain work of building, to the left-brain work of talking. She calls it "open the highway for the right to offer itself to the left" (p. 224). Regardless of which you choose, we like the aspect of 'inviting'—giving respect and power to the client, yet clearly indicating that a dialogue is desired with the purpose to understand the client's work. Usually even the quietest client is able to title the sandtray creation or give one feeling word.

The therapist–client dialogue in this post-creation phase needs further discussion, which we will provide in the following chapter.

Step Five: Sand Tray Cleanup

> To destroy a picture in the patient's presence would be to devalue a completed creation, to break the connection between the patient and his inner self, and the unspoken connection to the therapist. (Weinrib, 1983, p. 14)

This step may or may not be part of the session with the client. Once the sandtray scene and subsequent discussion have been completed, it is time to put the miniature figures away. Note that some clients will become so absorbed in the creation of the tray that it may be necessary for the therapist to give appropriate time warnings observing the end of the session is approaching. While it is important for the boundary of the session's time limit to be maintained, it is unfair to simply cut off a client in the middle of a sandtray creation. Clients often need a reflective time following the nonverbal expression of deep emotions. Depending on the client and the session it might be a 5-minute or 10-minute warning, with subsequent count-down as needed and appropriate.

Once the session is done, the dismantling of the sandtray scene should be done after the client has left the room. Leaving the sandtray intact honors and respects the client's work. There is another important perspective involved with dismantling the tray after the client has left. Just as in play therapy, where the play is the language and the toys are the words—in sandtray therapy, the miniature figures are the words. At a deeper level, they are the expression of the client's emotional life and inner self. We would not want to communicate with clients a message that their emotional expression needs to be "cleaned up" and is therefore unacceptable. While children and adolescents (adults, too!) need to learn to clean up after themselves, we do not view the dismantling of the sandtray to be related. It also is the dismantling of the metaphoric and symbolic work— the narrative of the client. We believe honoring this narrative is reflective of leaving the sandtray creation intact.

Dismantling the tray after the client leaves also allows the client to leave with the visual image of the scene in his or her mind. Many clients will continue to do their own processing and thinking about the imagery and metaphor of their sandtray during the time until the next session. Some clients will even continue to ponder the meaning of the tray, or items in the tray, for many weeks to follow. This is obviously a powerful extension of the therapy hour. Linda had an adult client who would come to a session weeks after a sandtray session and begin by saying, "Remember that horse? I know what it means!" and she would continue to relate the symbolic meaning for her and her current life situation. Even months after a particular sandtray session, this client would refer to "the horse" or other figures in her sandtray as a kind of shorthand to express her feelings or meaning of a situation. Powerful!

Some therapists will cover the clients' trays with a veil, to further communicate the message of honoring the clients' creation.

If there is still time remaining in the session and you or the client would like to do another tray, both people can dismantle the scene, returning the miniatures to their spots on the shelves. As a means of honoring the client's work, it is suggested that you allow the client to remove the first miniatures. The counselor may then offer, "I'll help," and assist in expediting the process. This allows the creator of the scene to be the one to initiate the dismantling the creation. Linda had a pre-adolescent who worked well in the sand tray and he liked doing several scenes in a single session. His anxiety, however, precluded him allowing himself the time to remove the miniature figures from the tray. He would simply swipe them all off to one end. While it resulted with a mound of figures by the end of the session, and a smaller and small space in which for him to build, it worked for him.

The counselor's perspective and purpose again determine how the remaining portion of the session is used. For example, a counselor may first have the client create a nondirected scene, followed with a directed one. This would be helpful for the client who needs time to feel comfortable with the media. However, some clients do better beginning with a directed scene first. This might be the anxious client or the "need-to-please" client. Interaction in a structured manner with the media allows an opportunity to, again, become comfortable with the media. Another option may be for the counselor to ask the client to say which type of work he/she would like to do—directed or nondirected.

Step Six: Documenting the Sandtray Therapy Session

Typically, photographs of the completed sandtray scenes are taken and placed in the client file. This should, of course, only be done with the client's permission, and can be included in the informed consent. These pictures can be invaluable for the therapist who desires to review the progress of a given client over a period of time. Additionally, this photographic chronology can be reviewed by the client and therapist in the assessment of progress and evaluation for termination.

One valuable way of wrapping up and terminating with a sandtray therapy client can be to go through a "slide show" of their trays, shown on the therapist's desktop monitor or laptop computer. This is a powerful way to achieve the therapeutic task at termination of summarizing the journey.

We used to use instant (Polaroid™) pictures, which were easily taken and then stapled to a session progress form. In this digital age, sharper and clearer images are available and can be printed out and attached, or the image inserted into, a session progress form. Using instant film or a 35-mm camera has gone the way of the 8-track tape. A digital photograph taken on one's smart phone or digital camera is more likely the method of documenting the trays. Awareness of cyber-hacking, storing in the Cloud, and other possible breeches of confidentiality remain an issue.

Another benefit of taking a picture of the client's tray is the assistance it provides for continued discussion in subsequent sessions. It is possible that one tray produces such rich material upon which to process, that an additional session or two is needed. Having the picture to view, for both the therapist and client, is invaluable.

A Note of Caution: If a picture is given to a client (especially a child client), it should be carefully screened by the sandtray therapist for the content of the sandtray scene. Protecting the client's confidentiality is always important.

Also, having the client take a picture of the scene from his or her perspective can also be very informative. The client's view can also add additional layers of meaning. We have done both types of photographs of a sandtray: the client's view and an overhead view by the clinician.

We have found that children especially enjoy having their picture taken with their sandtray. Copies of these pictures can also be used in termination with the client. Children who make a book (of drawings and/or text) of their time in counseling as a closure activity typically love having a picture or two added to their book. And the book can then become a nice transitional object at the conclusion of a therapeutic relationship.

Other therapists, seeking to keep costs under control (and having the requisite talent!) simply sketch the primary figures of the sandtray in appropriate rectangles on the session forms. This is often sufficient to keep the highlights. However, this does not allow for more thorough review—there are often aspects of the process and the tray, which at the time, may have seemed insignificant, but in review might be noticed as a beginning of a trend or repeated symbol.

Still other therapists, with profound respect for the amount of communication possible in a sandtray, prefer not to capture it in photographs. The concern is to maintain the confidentiality of the client from others who may later see the file. To these clinicians, the picture is equal to a verbatim transcript of a session, and thus could be overly intrusive. Documentation of the sessions, it is believed, should be the same as for any verbal session.

As with other therapeutic modalities, it may be helpful in the training and continued supervision process to videotape the sandtray therapy sessions. This should be done only with the appropriate authorization, and keeping in mind the need to balance the supervision benefits with the need to provide the client with a "free and protected space."

We have provided some sample clinical forms in Appendix A. We encourage the reader to develop a form that works in his or her setting and approach. Please feel free to adapt any of the forms in this book for your use.

6

Processing the Sandtray Therapy Session

Processing the scene in the sandtray can be an intensely powerful experience for both the client and the clinician. The clinician may have insights into the world of the client, based both on previous interactions with the client and from the content of the scene in the sandtray. Meanings or interpretations of the miniature figures and formations in the sandtray can be amazingly similar, regardless of the client's issues or age. While this tends to intrigue even the most "non-Jungian" of us, we would again caution against excessive interpretation. John Allan (1988) wisely advises: "The crux of Sandplay is not that it must be interpreted but that it must be witnessed respectfully" (p. 221).

There are many ways to process the tray with a client. As stated previously, the intention and purpose for using sandtray therapy with a specific client may well shape and direct the processing of the created tray. We will discuss several different approaches we have used. Certainly, this will not be all-inclusive. However, we hope this will provide the reader with some new or additional possibilities.

Processing sandtrays will also differ according to the therapist's theoretical orientation. This is one of our favorite aspects of the sandtray therapy process. It is truly cross-theoretical. For the Adlerian therapist, sandtray therapy is a wonderful lifestyle analysis tool (Sweeney, Minnix, & Homeyer, 2003); for the narrative therapist, it is an effective tool in assisting clients to tell their story; for the Jungian, it is the doorway to the psyche; for the cognitive therapist, it is a tool for exploring and disputing irrational beliefs; and for the family systems therapist, sandtray is a tool for exploring family of origin issues and communication dynamics. This list could obviously go on.

This chapter provides some practical questions to use during this process, briefly describes some case examples, and touches upon the assessment of progress in sandtray therapy. Specific suggestions for working with groups, couples, families, and integration of cognitive/structure techniques are in the following chapters.

WHO LEADS THE PROCESS?

Before discussing ways that we process the sandtray, we need to makes some comments about *who* in fact leads this process. Previously, we've talked about the fact that sandtray therapy is always a facilitative process, and can be directed or nondirected. Even when it is a structured exercise (see Chapters 7–9), we want the client to feel the safety and empowerment of a facilitator.

Having said this, when we ask clients to bring us into their world, we are asking them to be our tour guide. Caesar and Roberts (1991) talk about this process, with the therapists' role being tourists traveling on a journey with clients—and the clients being the tour guides. This is, in fact, the picture of empathy. We are the tourists being transported into the clients' world, as opposed to compelling them to enter ours.

In fact, we will often use this language—both in therapy and in sandtray therapy training—that the client is the *tour guide*, bringing us in and through their sandtray creations. This is particularly important in the process of family and group sandtray, where clients are guiding other family or group members through their own creations. When we ask clients to create a world or scene, it is only natural that they are the tour guide as we begin the process of exploring the sand tray creations.

USING THE METAPHOR

We would argue that it is important to keep the discussion within the metaphor or story of the tray. This provides the necessary distancing that the client may need in order to work through issues. This is a particular strength of sandtray therapy.

- The client may be able to introduce a difficult issue through the safety of a metaphorical sandtray scene. The client who needs this avenue of communication may not be able to introduce the same subject verbally—because of a lack of emotional and psychological safety—that is provided by the concreteness of the sandtray scene.
- The client may introduce therapeutic material without being aware of doing so. Only during the processing of the tray is "hidden" material revealed.
- The sandtray and its contents become the focus of the discussion rather than the client. With the focus removed from the client, the client is able to more freely discuss his or her issues.

The therapist should not, therefore, remove the safety of the metaphor and therapeutic distance of the sandtray process by direct interpretation. The purpose of using a projective and expressive medium is circumvented if the counselor is too directive or confrontive. Moon (2015), an art therapist, suggested:

> Affixing a specific diagnostic or psychological label to an artwork, which appears to be the ultimate end of interpretive events, leads to what I describe as imagicide (Moon, 2015). Imagicide is the intentional killing of an image through labeling it as one thing and thus restricting it. One may wonder what might motivate an art therapist to commit imagicide. Can imagicide be attributed to an art therapist's need to be perceived by others (employers or colleagues) as an "authority that analyzes and explains what images and artworks "really mean"? (Moon, 2015, p. 70)

These strong words apply to sandtray therapists who rob clients of their own interpretation by foisting the therapists' own view or interpretation of the sandtray creation and its contents.

ENLARGING THE MEANING

Enlarging the meaning, a play therapy technique, can be useful in processing sand trays. Enlarging the meaning takes the content or metaphor of the tray, and adds or enlarges meaning. When reflected (tentatively, so that the message can be either accepted or rejected) to the client, it frequently facilitates insight. This technique is based on the philosophical view that clients of all ages may be great perceivers but often poor interpreters.

Children, for example, take in a great deal of information, but can only interpret that information from their developmentally limited perspective. This results in the establishment of internalized misbeliefs about themselves and their world. Adults, likewise, take in information, but often continue to interpret it through their previously established misbeliefs. Clients, both children and adults, typically do not identify misbeliefs without assistance. This is the role of the counselor, through the use of responses that enlarge the meaning.

The first step to enlarging the meaning is to enter the client's world. This entails understanding the client's world from his or her perception. The counselor verbally reflects this to the client. Based on this understanding of the client's perception and adding to that the counselor's knowledge of the dynamics of the client's issues, the counselor can expand the meaning. This response facilitates that which we believe many clients cannot do alone—putting the clients' misbelief into words.

This opens the door to assist clients to challenge their misbeliefs; to avoid the emergence of new misbeliefs; to avoid reinforcement of previously held misbeliefs. Rather, the challenging of misbeliefs is facilitated by the insight provided by the counselor's use of enlarging the meaning.

Here is an example. Clients who have been victimized may minimize the intrapsychic or interpersonal damage resulting from this awful experience. Perhaps few (if any) people have believed their story. As their stories emerge and develop, the sandtray therapist can comment about this, often beginning with responses to the miniature(s):

- That must have been awful for "the miniature" to have experienced this.
- I wonder if anyone believed when "the miniature" told about what happened.
- Looks like it was so awful for "the miniature" that she or he never told anyone.
- This should never have happened to "the miniature."
- No one should feel this lonely.
- No one deserves what "the miniature" experienced.

EXCEPTIONS TO STAYING IN THE METAPHOR

The exception to staying within the metaphor of the sandtray would be when the client initiates making the connection between elements in the sandtray scene and his or her life situation. Clients who make this verbal connection are ready to do so. We trust clients will do so when they are ready. The counselor's need to prematurely push the client to make that connection will, we believe, interrupt the client's movement toward growth and healing. Few of us would argue that the purpose of therapy is to meet the needs of the client rather than the therapist.

In addition to the caution not to push clients prematurely, it is helpful to remember another dynamic. We need to be aware that clients inherently want to please therapists (and, children inherently want to please adults). Thus, for the therapist who is impatient or has an agenda, clients may well move to verbalizing issues before they are ready. A simple reminder to sandtray therapists—trust the process!

PROCESSING THE SESSION

Processing a sandtray with an individual client is generally pretty much the same regardless if the individual client is a child, teenager, or adult. Obviously, appropriate developmental considerations should be taken into account.

Where to Begin

One approach is to begin with the global view and work toward the more detailed focus. This would begin with a discussion of the entire scene, and then discuss the sections or parts, ending with the individual miniature figures and items.

Regardless of how one begins, if the client has been standing and moving around during the creation of the scene and is still standing, invite the client to have a seat. This communicates to the client that you want him/her to be comfortable. It also communicates that you want to spend some time discussing the scene. Pull both chairs up to the side of the sandtray for easy viewing. Sit on the side from which the scene is constructed. Most, but not all clients, will build with an easily identified front and back of the scene. Having said this—don't assume! Let the client identify it, if it is unclear. There will also be clients who want to be able to look at the sandtray therapist across the tray, and not have to turn aside from the tray to look at the therapist. So be attuned and ask to clarify if needed.

Some clients will want to touch and even pick up items from the sandtray as they talk. Other clients may run their fingers through the sand. Remember that this tactile contact with the sand is therapeutic and may be necessary for the client who needs to self-soothe while discussing the content of the tray. This results in an ability to increase self-regulation and learn the skill to do so while processing difficult content.

Case Example: Adult Female

The client is a 40-year-old female and this is her first sandtray, seen in Figure 6.1. She had been in therapy with Linda for approximately 40 sessions before introduction of the sand tray. Some art techniques had been successfully used in previous sessions. The client lived alone, was self-isolated, and had frequently been suicidal. Her therapy had focused on her childhood sexual abuse, the death of her mother when she was a preadolescent, the recent death of her father (about two years prior), and sexual identity issues. An only child with no extended family, she was virtually alone. She has several

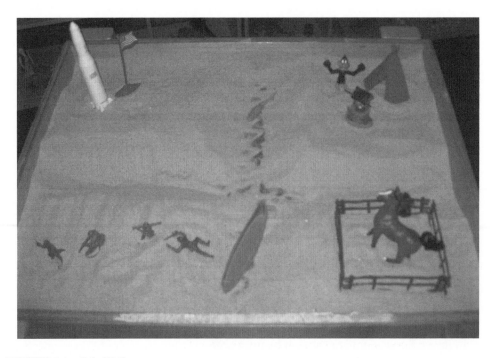

FIGURE 6.1 "My life."

years of her childhood that she cannot remember. We met regularly in the sandttray room, so she we familiar with the materials. For this session, the prompt for building the tray was "Build a scene of your world" using the nondirective approach.

"What Is the Title?"

This is an easy beginning question. The very title that a client gives to her scene or world may provide invaluable insight into how the client views self and interaction with her world. As mentioned in the previous chapter, even the most reticent client is able to come up with a title. It might be as brief as "My Life." Or, it may be more of a summary statement about the creation, such as, "My Life: What It's Like Now and How I Want It to Be in the Future."

How you phrase this question is important. Asking a closed question such as, "Would you like to title your picture?" may result in the client telling you, "No!" Unless you are willing to accept that answer, word it more appropriately.

"Tell Me about It."

This is the invitation to have the client tell about the entire sandtray, the global view. If the client responds with some hesitation or resistance, you may need to provide encouragement. A response of "I don't know what it means, it's just a picture," may be responded with, "Perhaps you can just make up a story about it." The metaphorical meanings will still emerge in the telling of the story. Allow as much free narrative as possible, using facilitative responses and attending skills to let the client know you are paying attention and understanding. When the client is done, respond with a short summary of what has been told to you.

Client:	Sandtray Therapist:
Well, this is about my life. Here (pointing to the upper right scene) is how I am today. See, this is me, happy. (pointing at the Donald Duck™ figure with arms raised)	
	You're happy here.
Yea, then . . . I put in the horse, 'cause I've always liked horses. The river separates this side with my future. The soldiers represent my hope to be back with the Army Reserves.	*Um-m-m.*
	Okay.
The rocket ship . . . well, I've always wanted to explore and . . . go to different places . . . Well, that kinda represents that.	*So, you have three scenes. This side is how you are now, feeling good about what is going on. Across the river, which is your future, are two scenes. This one (pointing to the soldiers) is about your goal to be back in the Reserves and the other is about further in the future. Right?*
Right	

In this example, the client has briefly introduced each section when giving an overall explanation of the tray. Discussion of the various scenes is the logical next step.

"Tell Me More about What's Happening in This Scene."

This will provide the client with the opportunity to be more detailed in the explanation of each scene. This also communicates the therapist's interest and investment in the process. During the explanation and discussion of each scene, the client may begin to self-interpret the meaning of some of the miniatures. Others may not. Asking questions to clarify or obtain additional information is appropriate.

Client:	Sandtray Therapist:
The tee-pee is my house. You didn't have one like I really want to have so I picked that one. And this is me. (Donald Duck™ with raised arms.)	
	"Tell me about the way she's standing. (I use "she" because the client is female, although she picked Donald.)
Well, it's like a victory stance.	
	She is feeling pretty good about herself. She feels like she's won! (As I look at her, she smiles a bit sheepishly.)
Yes. It feels good! (Her sheepish smile grows to a broad smile.)	
That's kinda like what we do in here. (Her face becomes sober.) *We lower the bucket down and it comes back up full of black, oily, smelly stuff. Then we pour it out, and talk about it until it's all gone. Then we put the bucket back down for some more.*	*Tell me about this* (pointing at the wishing well). (Wow—I was impressed! I expected her to talk about cool, fresh, reviving water—my image of the wishing well. Instead, her image was that of dealing with her past life events and her "out-of-awareness." The wishing well remained a powerful metaphor for the remainder of our work together.) *You've really worked hard in here. You have been willing to look at a lot of hard stuff.*
Yeah, I know. (She smiles sheepishly.)	
	So, this is how you are now. Tell me about . . . (and I move on to another scene)

There is no need to rush this process. If there is quality interaction occurring, simply allow it to continue and unfold. It would not be unusual to discuss one section of the tray in depth for the remainder of the session. Once all the scenes are discussed move on to the next level, which is to ask about specific figures.

Clients can usually describe why they put a certain miniature or item in their scene. As noted above, my client talked about why she picked the cartoon character to represent her. Not because she thought of herself as cartoonish (although she still had a long way to go for a positive self-image), but because of the victor stance. She shared that she placed the wishing well in her scene because she just "liked the looks of it." It was only when we were talking about the scene that she reported that the metaphor of her dealing with her dark past in counseling "came to her." This is a common experience with clients. Initially they "just know" that an item should be in the scene. Only later, while discussing the scene, do they surprise even themselves with the item's special meaning. Later in the session, after we had talked about most of the contents of the scene, I asked about the river. While initially I would have indicated the organization of the tray had two halves, divided by a river, and each half had two scenes, it does, in fact, have *five* scenes. The river is a section as well. She had not brought it up, so I asked her the following question:

"I Notice . . . (Pointing at the Shark in the River). Tell Me about It."

Client:	Sandtray Therapist:
Well, see this (pointing at the river) *is in the way of getting to the future.*	
	. . . and the shark?
Yeah! The shark can kill you!	
Yes.	(So quiet I can hardly hear her) *. . . before you even get there.* (An enlarging-the-meaning response.)

Leaving the Sandtray Intact

The continued power of the sandtray image has been mentioned previously. This is the primary reason not to dismantle the scene before the client leaves the room—to maintain the scene in the client's mind. The client who constructed this tray came in several weeks after making this tray, bubbling over with excitement. "I figured it out!" she said. She went on to relate that she realized the reason for the horse in the fenced area. She stated it wasn't just that this horse, which should be free, was being kept penned in for the convenience of its owner (this had been her previous explanation of that part of the tray). Now, she realized *she* was the horse: An animal that should be free and wild, allowed to be what it was created to be. Not broken by men, to be ridden and under their control, used for their convenience. She, too, had been broken and ridden by men, for their convenience, and under their control (raped and molested); not allowed to be free as she was created to be. This insight finally gave her the freedom to be angry and she began grieving over what had been taken from her. Until that session, she had never been able to fully articulate the depths of what the sexual abuse and assualt had done to her. The metaphor of the horse held her pain and loss. I believe this was the day I fell in love with the power of sandtray therapy.

> Not infrequently patients report that they consciously carry the image of the sand tray in their minds. They may focus on and re-experience some part of a picture they have made, or change it, or they may make imaginary new pictures which they often then create in reality at the next opportunity (Weinrib, 1983, p. 52).

ANOTHER OPTION: FOCUS PROCESSING

It is also possible to move from the client titling the tray to the counselor asking specific questions about individual miniature figures. The client, in the above example, had a very organized world. When she finished building her world, it was clear that there were specific scenes with apparent connections. The global approach is well suited to that type of tray.

Other clients, or perhaps the example client at another time, may build a disorganized, chaotic, or empty world. These sandtrays are not as easily discussed using the global approach. The following approach may be more appropriate.

Focus Processing

1. Ask the client to title the tray.
2. Ask the client to describe the overall scene.
   Again, allow as much free narrative as possible. It is always best to provide the opportunity for the client to communicate his or her understanding of the tray. What may look like a chaotic or empty scene may have a different meaning to the client.
3. Invite the client to discuss specific figures.
   How do you decide which miniature to ask the client about first? This is a key question! As indicated in an earlier chapter, the counselor takes a moment to respond to the completed scene in the tray. Use your response to the tray as a beginning.
   a. Does one miniature stand out for some reason? Larger than the rest? Smaller? Different? Proximity? That would be a useful place to start.
   b. How do you affectively respond to the tray? Does a certain miniature or its placement evoke some emotion? Another useful place to begin: Resonating with the emotion in the tray with the therapist maintaining that 'bridge' and connecting with the client's emotional resonating as well.

1. Title the tray
2. Describe the entire tray
3. Discuss specific miniature figures

c. It is often helpful to ask clients which miniature symbol represents them; however, we suggest that this inquiry be carefully worded. We would *not* suggest asking the client: "*Where* are you in here?" This obviously assumes that the client has placed herself in the tray, which may be an unfair assumption, and may result in the client picking out a miniature in order to satisfy the therapist, rather than it being a true representation. If clients have not addressed this issue in their initial explanation of the tray, it is better to simply ask: "Are you in here?"

d. If it feels clinically appropriate and timely, the therapist can ask: "If you were in this scene, is there a miniature—either in the tray already or still on the shelves—that might represent you?" (This also invites the client to add another item to represent self, if desired.)

e. If the client does not offer any information on this, the therapist can consider which miniature may represent the client.

f. It can also be helpful to ask the client if there are other person(s) represented in the tray. It should not be assumed that a client's partner, child, friend, perpetrator, and so on will automatically be included among the miniature items.

g. *Which miniature has the most power?* It might be the largest item, or perhaps the monster miniature, or the army tank—remember, however, that clients may have their own and different insight.

4. Invite the client to give voices to the miniature figures.
   What would the miniature say about the scene? Their role in the scene? Their relationship with another miniature? To the client? It may be helpful to initiate a dialogue between miniatures, similar to the empty chair technique or puppet play therapy.

5. Intuitive nature or meaning of the miniature figures.
   Understanding some of the typical meanings of miniatures provides the counselor with another source of possible questions or a place from which to "springboard" into the discussion of the client's tray.

6. Observe client's interaction with the miniatures and media.
   While the client was building the scene in the tray, what did you notice? Reluctance to include a miniature that was finally used? Touching, stroking of a miniature, hard to put it down? Avoidance of a particular miniature or category of miniatures?

7. Invite the client to proceed with the action.
   We noted previously that children will often play out scenes in the sandtray, as opposed to creating a single scene. This process can be very revealing and therapeutically beneficial. It is possible to ask a client, "What might happen next?" Or, "What might this (figure) say to this (other figure)?"

Two important notes: (a) While some therapists and books point to the symbolic meaning of toys and miniatures, it is unfair to foist these meanings onto a client's creation. The fact that they used several dinosaur miniatures may have no other meaning than having recently watched a Hollywood film. (b) Do *not* touch the miniatures in the tray. This is unfairly intrusive. If you'd like to point to miniatures during the processing of the tray, be sure not to make contact with your finger.

These are some possible ways to connect with the client through the sandtray process. It provides a structure through which the client can share his or her meaning of the sandtray scene. It also provides the counselor with ways to assist the client in exploring possible deeper meanings.

Case Example 2: Young Male Adolescent

This client was a 13-year-old boy who was referred for therapy because he had responded to his own sexual victimization by victimizing a younger foster girl in his home. His parents were foster parents, and he was referred to Daniel for therapy due to the obvious situation, but also because of his increasing behavioral disruption at home and in school.

Before discussing the sandtrays pictured, it may be helpful to briefly describe a mother–son session involving this client prior to these individual trays. I had requested to see the entire family (father, mother, and two sons), but only the mother consented to come in (for one time only). She essentially wanted her son to be seen, to get better, and for the therapist to "certify" to the local child welfare agency that the family was "safe" to again be a foster family (needless to say, the foster daughter had been removed).

When the mother and her son arrived, I asked that they create a tray together. A dynamic that occurred repeatedly in the tray construction involved the son either placing or asking permission to place spiders, snakes, and lizards in the tray. Each time the mother would say no, or would remove the items placed by her son. The mother placed a bride and groom in the tray, to which the son asked if it represented her and his father. When she responded that they did, the son promptly placed a tank in the tray and "shot" the bride and groom. This dynamic repeated itself several times.

The metaphorical meaning behind this activity seemed clear. The mother wanted her son "fixed"; she did not want to discuss family dynamics. The son's placement of "creepy crawly things" (as his mother described them) was a metaphor for his need to deal with some of the ugly issues in his life; the mother's removal of these things was a picture of her unwillingness to face these difficult issues. This was consistent with her verbal messages before, during, and after this session.

The tray pictured in Figure 6.2 is representative of many sandtray creations that this client constructed in the earlier stages of therapy. It involves a battle—a battle in

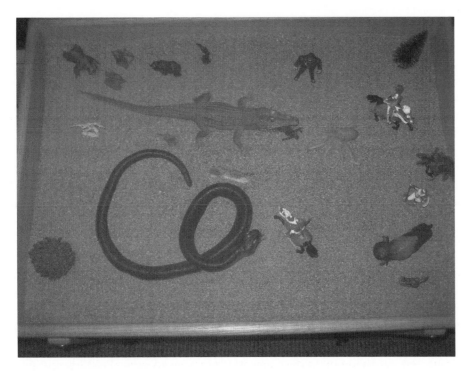

FIGURE 6.2   "Rumble of the earth"

which no one wins. This was certainly reflective of the client's emotional perception of his situation, which was indeed a place of great conflict from which he felt there was no escape. As the therapy continued, victories emerged from the battle, and provision made for escape.

A very clear projection emerged in the sandtray scenes of this client, which is reflected in this tray. You will note that there are two large figures—the snake and the alligator. As noted in Chapter 4, it can be helpful to have a few sand tray items that are disproportionately large. When a client is exploring victimization issues in the tray, large predatory creatures are effective metaphors for the emotionally (and physically) overwhelming experiences of being victimized. Two neighborhood adolescents had molested this client, and it was very typical to see two large predatory creatures in most of his early trays. Later in the therapy process, he even named the two creatures with the same names as the offenders, not knowing that I knew the names from the intake information.

"What Is the Title of This Scene?"

The title he gave the tray was "Rumble of the Earth." This descriptive title speaks of the client's perception of the trauma he experienced, as well as the emotional aftermath. In addition to the picture of the rumbling of an earthquake (definitely an out-of-control experience), there is also the conflict of a *rumble*—an adolescent gang fight. This is essentially what the client experienced when victimized by neighborhood teens.

"What Is Happening in Here?"

The client described the scene as "people from the future fighting in medieval times." You will notice from the picture that there are both modern soldiers and medieval knights engaged in the struggle. Despite what would seem to be an advantage—modern soldiers with modern weaponry—there are no victors. The client is expressing that despite the resources he had, he was nevertheless victimized. It was a traumatic experience beyond his control.

"Are You in This Scene?"

The client said that the knight fighting the snake represented him. Recalling that there were no victors in this struggle, it is noted that the client chose the large phallic predatory creature in which to be engaged within a losing battle.

"What Has the Most Power in Here?"

I choose to use the word *what* instead of *whom*, so as to not limit the client's choice. This client stated that the alligator had the most power. It is interesting to note that he chose one of the two predators, but not the one with which he was engaged. The client is feeling empowered in the session by the opportunity to process his issues in a nonverbal manner, but does not feel ready or willing to directly engage at this point.

The tray, Figure 6.3, shows a continuation of the battle theme, but has some notable differences. There are the two intruders, who are depicted in the tanks, but they are advancing upon a well-defended fort. One of the key advantages of sandtray therapy is that through the metaphors of the play, the client is able to 'manage' that which was 'unmanageable.' When in the midst of chaos and trauma, the lack of control is particularly emotionally impacting. The ability to engage in a projective and expressive medium allows the client to regain some of the control lost in the life experiences precipitating the behavioral and emotional symptoms leading to a referral for therapy.

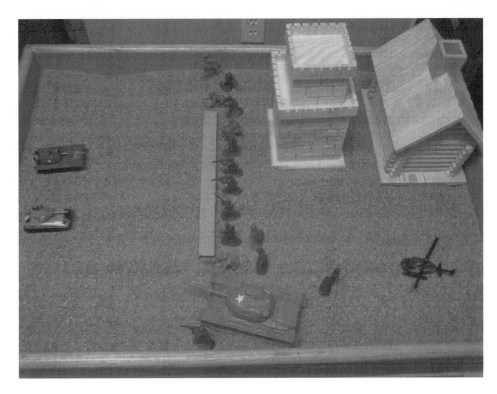

FIGURE 6.3   "Defending the fort"

"What Is the Title of This Scene?"

The client entitled this tray "Defending the Fort." As noted, the two intruders are present, albeit noticeably smaller than in the previous picture. The perpetrators have less power in this scene, and the client has greater defenses.

"What Is Happening in Here?"

The client proceeded to describe how the two tanks were attempting to attack the fort, but that the fort was too heavily protected to fall to defeat. When I asked him if he was in the scene, he said that he was inside the fort building, and that we were not going to get hurt this time. It is interesting to note the helicopter parked next to the fort, which may metaphorically represent a means of escape.

The client is expressing several things in this tray. He is, as noted above, attempting to 'manage' in the fantasy of the sandtray that which was not manageable in the reality of his abuse. He is also displaying the development of insight and coping skills with which to frame his traumatizing experience. As the therapy process moved in this direction, many of the negative externalizing behaviors noted by his mother in school and at home were beginning to subside.

ANOTHER OPTION: REARRANGING

Following the creation of their sandtray, clients may need to rearrange, or change, what they have created in the tray. This may be a reflection of the global change or rearranging needed in the lives of clients, or the need to process a specific situation, that promotes safety and control in this circumstance.

This rearranging may occur in a self-initiated way by clients themselves, or may be an offer extended by the therapist. Clients may add or remove miniatures, which is certainly acceptable as part of the creation process. In fact, this may be an indication that the creative process is not yet complete. Even when clients indicate that they have completed their sandtray creation, they may make changes. We have experienced clients make changes in the tray all the way until the end of the therapeutic hour. Remember, this is the clients' creation—they are free to make as many changes as they would like!

The sandtray therapist may want to extend an offer to the client that changing or rearranging is an option. This may in fact be part of a structured sandtray intervention (see Chapter 7). However, it is crucial to be mindful that clients may be hypersensitive to criticism (perhaps even a perfectionist, like some therapists . . .)—and any suggestion that something might be *wrong* with their tray—through an offer to change or rearrange—may be damaging. It is therefore important to communicate to clients that the world they have created is acceptable as it is. It is merely an option that a client may take. Offering this to a client is essentially up to the therapist, if clinical intuition or therapeutic plan leads to this.

There are other considerations when clients choose to rearrange their sandtray creations. First, it may be appropriate to dialog with clients about the differences between the "first" tray and the "rearranged" tray. We should be cognizant that both creations have significant meaning, and that the client's choice to rearrange (and, the process of rearrangement) has equally significant meaning. Second, we do not want to rob clients of the opportunity to fully experience their initial creation before the *possible invitation* to rearrange. Be sensitive to the clients' emotional investment in their initial creation.

ASSESSING PROGRESS AND READINESS FOR TERMINATION

The assessment of progress in sandtray therapy is essentially similar to any other therapeutic modality, except that the therapist has the additional input of the sandtray process. It is important to look beyond the amelioration of symptoms to the resolution of intrapsychic conflict.

There is frequently an evident developmental progression of the sandtray therapy process. John Allan (1988) discusses common stages in the sandtray process with children, which we believe is helpful in assessing the progress of all clients. The first stage is *chaos*, in which clients may dump miniatures into the sand, often without any apparent deliberate selection. The chaos evident in the sand may be reflective of the chaos and emotional turmoil in the life of the client(s). Most marriage and family therapists are familiar with the 'dumping' of issues that families and couples do in the counseling process.

The next stage described is *struggle*, in which there may be overt or covert conflict, often "battle" scenes. At the beginning of this creative process, often the two (or more) sides in the fight will annihilate each other. In other words, the world depicts a no-win situation. Although the scene may reflect one side winning (e.g., a dominant partner over an unassertive, compliant partner), it really isn't a win–lose situation, it is a lose–lose situation. We have often found that in the early stages of sandtray therapy (with children and adults), that no one survives these battles or accidents.

With positive progress, and the process of building relationship and communication, the sandtray therapy moves to the third stage, which Allan describes as *resolution*, where life seems to be 'getting back to normal.' There is more order and balance in the tray, miniatures are deliberately selected and carefully placed, and the clients see themselves in the trays, often in helpful and egalitarian roles. This is usually a sign that termination is appropriate, with the confirmation of external positive reports.

It is important in the evaluation of therapeutic progress to assess issues both within the sandtray therapy and outside of the sessions. Some questions to consider regarding the sandtray construction and processing in session include the following:

- Does the sandtray reflect less dependence and more autonomy?
- Is there an increase in the amount and quality of verbalization in therapy?
- Is there evidence that the client is developing greater insight and an internal sense of self-evaluation?
- Are the miniature figures placed with a greater degree of deliberation and order?
- Can the client more readily identify self, others, themes, and metaphors in the sandtray?
- Is the client's affective response to the sandtray process more predictable and congruent?
- Is the therapist's affective response to the client's tray reasonable and congruent with the client?
- Is there an absence of or minimal use of buried objects in the sand?
- Are barriers (e.g., fences, walls, etc.) used appropriately (reflection of healthy, as opposed to rigid or diffuse boundaries)?
- Are there fewer of Bühler's other clinical indicators (see Chapter 11)?

When assessing progress, indicators should be seen both inside and outside of the sandtray therapy room. We should expect to see increased levels of independence in therapy and at home, work, or school. We should also expect changes that are more global and generalized in the life of the client. Sweeney (1997) suggested several changes in the life of the client that should be evident in play sessions, as well as generalized beyond the therapeutic setting:

- Increased ability to solve problems.
- Increased verbalization (although this should not be an agenda for the therapist).
- Greater willingness to experiment and explore.
- Increased self-worth and self-confidence and corresponding decreased shame and self-deprecation.
- Decreased anxiety and depression.
- Increased ability to organize and order things and corresponding decreased chaotic thinking and behavior.
- Increased ability to express emotions and tolerate other people's expression of emotions.
- Decreased aggression.
- Decreased fear of confrontation and corresponding increased willingness to negotiate.
- Increased willingness to give and receive nurture.
- Increased tolerance of frustration.
- Increased willingness to seek assistance.
- Increased ability to make decisions.
- Changes in creative expression, including stories, artwork, etc.

(Sweeney, 1997, p. 146)

As noted in the previous chapter, it can be very helpful to review the progress of a sandtray client through a review of the pictures or slides of the trays completed over the course of therapy. Themes and metaphors can be discussed, as well as the changes in these throughout the course of intervention. The insight that clients frequently display in this review process is remarkable, and can be a way of evaluating readiness for termination and a way of concluding the therapeutic process with a client.

ONE LAST COMMENT

In processing sandtray creations, we would encourage sandtray therapists to be (much) more reflective than interrogative. Since a distinct advantage of expressive interventions is that they allow clients to express self through a nonverbally bound intervention, it is important to not draw clients back into verbalization through questions—which inherently call for a cognitive response. Thus, if inquiries can be rephrased into reflective statements, we stay with one of the basic purposes and rationale for doing sandtray therapy. Easier said than done, we know!

7

Integrating Sandtray Therapy with a Variety of Approaches and Techniques

While the primary benefit of sandtray therapy lies in the intrapsychic and interpersonal safety created by its expressive and projective nature, there is great potential to adapt both new and established techniques into the sandtray process. In fact, it is the very safety that is created in the expressive and projective elements of sandtray therapy that lends itself to such adaptation. With the reminder that it continues to be important to honor the client's developmental level, there are numerous structured therapeutic techniques that can be used to educate and provide insight for clients.

It may seem incongruent to combine sandtray with structured techniques—for example, solution-focused interventions. However, we would argue that this is a natural fit that has great potential. Cognitive and solution-focused techniques often call for responses that involve cognition and abstract thinking—fundamentally a verbal response. These interventions can actually find broader application when combined with an expressive intervention that does not begin with a required verbal response.

There are as many possible adaptations as there are existing and developing techniques. This chapter will consider a few, with hopes that readers will use their natural creativity as sandtray therapists to develop more. We remind readers to integrate new techniques with their understanding of therapeutic conceptualization (theory) and the therapeutic process (skills and session dynamics) with existing research for the overall benefit of the client. Obviously, therapists should have training in the following theories and interventions, as well as training in sandtray therapy.

RATIONAL-EMOTIVE BEHAVIOR THERAPY (REBT)

REBT takes the approach that emotional, behavioral, and relational problems stem not from events, but one's perception of the events. As such, the focus of REBT is upon the irrational beliefs held by the client (Ellis, 2008). The classic model developed by Ellis is the A-B-C model, which was later expanded to A-B-C-D-E. Essentially, the *A*ctivating event does not cause the emotional or behavioral *C*onsequence, but rather the *B*eliefs that are held by the person are the causal factors.

The intervention is, therefore, to *D*ispute the irrational beliefs, so that the *E*ffect is the reduction or elimination of the negative consequences. This is typically a verbal therapeutic process. However, this can be adapted to the sandtray therapy process. In a series of sandtray prompts, for example:

■ **A (Activating event):** "Please make a sandtray about a situation where you got angry."

■ **B (Beliefs):** "Make a sandtray about what you told yourself about this situation."
■ **C (Consequences):** "What about what this anger was like?"
■ **D (Dispute):** "I wonder if there is a different way of responding? Could you question your own angry thoughts? Make a tray of another way of looking at the situation."
■ **E (Effect):** "What would be your preferred way to respond? Can you make a tray of what this would look like? If you made a tray of what you can change, what should you expect/accept? Can you make a tray about this?"

This could be a series of separate trays, or a continuation of one tray, with changing scenes. For the client who has a challenging time verbalizing the A-B-C-D-E process, the sandtray can provide an effective alternative.

"PAIN GETTING BETTER" TECHNIQUE

Mills and Crowley (1986) proposed a three-part art intervention, called the "Pain Getting Better" technique. They have their child clients draw three pictures: (1) a picture of the pain, (2) a picture of the pain "all better," and (3) a picture of what will help picture number one change to picture number two. This can be nicely adapted for sandtray therapy, particularly for those who are less confident in their artistic ability.

Clients are asked to create three sand trays, corresponding to the instructions of the art technique. It is possible to have clients do three sections in a single tray (using dowels—see Chapter 8—to demark areas in the sand would be facilitative for this technique in one tray), but it seems more helpful to provide the separation that is often needed psychologically. These trays, which can be used with clients of all ages, help clients to not only project the pain, but also consider that life can indeed get better. Mills and Crowley (1986) describe some of the benefit:

> First, they help the child disconnect and contain the pain by transforming it into an image on paper. . . . Second, giving the pain a tangible image gives the child a sense of know-ing what she is dealing with—of moving from the unknown to the known. . . . A third purpose of the drawings is to help facilitate a switchover in sensory systems. . . . Drawing what the pain looks like helps activate other parts of the brain that diffuse attention and provide a wealth of helpful resources. The fourth purpose of the drawings is a powerful one of implication. By asking the child to draw how the pain would look "all better," the therapist is implying that "all better" does exist. (pp. 178–179)

These same benefits are transferable into the tray using similar visual attributes. The texture of the sand and figures add another helpful dimension.

SOLUTION-FOCUSED "MIRACLE QUESTION"

Solution-focused techniques can also be adapted well for use in the sandtray therapy process (Nims, 2007; Taylor, 2009). A specific directive technique that can be used in the sandtray is similar to the solution-focused "miracle question" (de Shazer, 1988), which serves to facilitate clients conceptualizing options, as well as a world beyond their current pain.

Traditionally, this might sound like: "If you woke up tomorrow, and sometime during the night a miracle happened and the problem that brought you here today was solved just like that, how would you know it happened? What would it look like?" These are fabulous questions that focus not only on the absence of the presenting problem, but also on imagining a future that is positive and ideal. Like many structured techniques, however, the miracle question calls for considerable abstract thinking, this may be too challenging for the client to verbalize.

The simple adaption would be this prompt: "If you woke up tomorrow, and sometime during the night a miracle happened and the problem that brought you here today was solved just like that, I wonder what that might look like? Could you make a sandtray of this? I wonder what your tray would be like, knowing this had happened?"

OTHER SOLUTION-FOCUSED QUESTIONS

There are a number of other solution-focused questions (de Shazer & Dolan, 2007) that can be adapted for use in the sandtray. Rather than asking for a verbal response, therapists ask clients to create sand trays that depict the answers, followed by verbal discussion. Some possible prompts are as follows:

- "Please make a tray that shows the last time this was *not* a problem."
- "This challenge could be a lot bigger—please make a tray about how you've kept this from getting to be a bigger problem."
- "If someone were making a movie about you having resolved this problem and the director yelled 'Cut' (stopping the filming) what would your life look like?"
- "Make a tray showing what you see down the road for yourself after this is resolved."
- "How will you even know that this is resolved? Can you make a tray on what this looks like?"
- "This past week—when you chose *not* to [argue, get depressed, act out]—what was it like? Show me in the tray what that would look/feel like."
- "This past week—when you chose to [argue, get depressed, act out]—what was it like? Show me in the tray what that would look/feel like."
- "Can you make a tray on what you might be doing, if you were to 'act as if' there was no problem? Show me what that would look like."
- "When you were dealing with this challenge a little better than you are right now, I'm wondering what that looked like. Could you make a tray of that on this side of the tray? Then on the other side, make a scene on what you might need to do in order to get back there."
- "If someone threw you a victory parade after you've journeyed though this, what would the parade be like?"
- "If your partner/friend/family member was here and making a tray about you, what would it look like?"
- "If I were making a sandtray to describe you—what kind of a tray would I make about you?"
- "If you picked a miniature to represent you and another to represent the challenge that brought you into counseling, what would these be? If you picked one or more miniatures to represent what it would take to subdue the one you chose to represent the challenge, what would these be?"
- "When things are moving in the right direction, what will that look like? Please make a tray showing this. Who will be the first person in your life to notice? What miniature would you select for this person? Place that person/image in the tray, too."
- "Make a tray on what is happening right now that you'd like to continue happening. What might you add to the tray to make this happen more frequently?"
- "If you could pick a miniature to represent me (the therapist), and how I might help—or, change what I've been doing—what figure would you choose?"

There are many other possible questions, and these are questions that clients may be able to answer verbally. For those clients who struggle to respond or for those clients whose answers are quick, brief, or shallow, sandtray therapy provides an alternative forum for response and process.

MOTIVATIONAL INTERVIEWING (MI)

In the *Motivational Interviewing* (MI) process (see Miller & Rollnick, 2002), there are four general principles, including: 1) express empathy; 2) develop discrepancy; 3) roll with resistance; and 4) support self-efficacy. For clients who are challenged with verbally engaging in the process, is it possible to express empathy, focus on discrepancies, roll with resistance, and support the self-efficacy with the sandtray miniatures, and then make the transition to the clients? Boyd-Franklin, Cleek, Wofsy and Mundy (2013) argue that while many clients feel shamed by their behaviors, MI avoids a shaming approach, suggesting: "The process of developing discrepancy recognizes that within each human being there are parts that want to change and parts that do not" (p. 119). We would suggest that the combination that MI honors in this ambivalence combines well with the therapeutic distance provided by sandtray therapy.

In Miller and Rollnick (2013) several questions are suggested in the MI practice:

1. "Why would you want to make this change?"
2. "How might you go about it in order to succeed?"
3. "What are the three best reasons for you to do it?"
4. "How important is it for you to make this change, and why?"
5. "So what do you think you'll do?"

(p. 11)

Could these questions be posed to sandtray miniature figures? For example, after the client has chosen a miniature to represent self [or, perhaps someone else, if the identification of self is too threatening]—asking the client: "Why would (this miniature) want to make this change" or "How might (this miniature) go about making this change, so that she might succeed?"

ROLE-PLAYING

A technique that is used with many theoretical approaches is role-playing. Using role-playing and drama therapy techniques in the sandtray therapy context is a natural fit. Simulation provides an effective means for learning skills, exploring relationships, and building self-awareness. Through the projective process of using miniatures, greater safety is created when approaching evocative material. There is stimulation in simulation, but safety in the tray.

An example of role-playing in the tray is the use of the Gestalt empty chair technique. Typically, this involves the client interacting with an absent person imaginably seated in the empty chair. Usually, the client will sit opposite the empty chair, and may switch positions in the role-play process. The therapist may assume the role of a coach, to assist the client, or may give voice to the empty chair. In sandtray therapy, the client simply selects miniature figures to represent self and the absent person. We have found it easier for clients to have a conversation between miniature figures than speak to an empty chair. If desired, the therapist can join the conversation in the form of a third miniature. We recommend having the client select this figure as well. This might be an initial step before moving to the empty chair. The level of control and 'smallness' of the miniature figures can provide the initial practice in a safer container. Then, the more transitional empty chair could be the next step in the therapeutic process. As we mention so often throughout this book-intentionality and purposefulness.

Clients can tell their story through an active sandtray, with the miniature figures taking on various roles. It is often safer for a client to narrate a scene through the miniatures engaged in domestic violence than directly verbalizing it. Staying with this scenario, the therapist can brainstorm with the client about planning and implementing a safety plan, using the miniature figures to act this out.

This psycho-educational dynamic of role-playing in the sandtray is invaluable. For the child or adolescent with poor peer relational skills, role-plays in the sandtray can be a great place to start, prior to the needed group therapy intervention. After clients tell their story through the action of miniatures in the tray, the therapist can inquire: "If this had turned out the way you wanted, could you make another tray of what that would look like?" Even if the situation involves a school-bullying incident and the client plays out a scene of violent retribution, the therapist can explore alternative solutions through the sandtray.

A variation of this may be to offer a suggestion like: "If your best friend was there to help you in this situation, what would he or she do?" If no one comes to mind for the client, or in fact if no one like this even exists for the client: "If you had a best friend, what would he or she be like? What miniature would you select to represent him or her?" As therapists, we know about the crucial importance of social support. While it may seem that this intervention could remind clients of their loneliness—and it could—it also gives the therapist a better picture of what the client needs, and assists in the development of a comprehensive treatment plan.

Role-playing can be directed by the client or by the therapist. It is certainly empowering for clients to be the directors and choreographers of the process, but it may be necessary for the therapist to initiate a drama or role-play for instructive and informative purposes or because the clients' anxiety has become overwhelming for them.

MINDFULNESS

As sandtray therapists and counselors, we look to move away from simply symptom reduction. In the same way, mindfulness, described by Hick and Bien (2010) as "focusing attention, being aware, intentionality, being nonjudgmental, acceptance, and compassion" (p. 5) looks to help clients acknowledge reality, accept circumstances, and develop healthier and more flexible intra- and inter-personal relationships with self and others. There are a myriad of mindfulness exercises, many of which can be adapted to sandtray therapy.

Many approaches to mindfulness focus on meditative techniques and stress reduction. For example, Kabat-Zinn (1990) formulated one of the first mindfulness-based interventions with his development of mindfulness-based stress reduction. One example of a mindfulness intervention that can be adapted for sandtray therapy is the *STOP* exercise (Stahl & Goldstein, 2010). This consists of teaching clients the following elements:

- **S:** stop, and interrupt your 'automatic pilot'—this begins with concentrating on the present moment.
- **T:** take a breath, and focus on your experience of breathing out and breathing in.
- **O:** openness to observation—connecting to your in-the-moment experience, considering what you are feeling, hearing, sensing, seeing, and even thinking.
- **P:** proceed, reconnecting with your surroundings and current activities.

Sandtray therapists may teach these concepts while clients are running their fingers through the sand, a very sensory and grounding experience. This can also involve the use of wet sand. Clients can also reinforce this teaching while holding a miniature figure representing them. The therapist can 'coach' the miniatures in the presence of the clients, or the clients can coach the miniature representing self, or other miniatures. This can be like the child who, as a part of playing, sets up a classroom of stuffed animals and takes on the role of teacher.

Additionally, a client can be asked to create a tray around the issue of how a presenting challenge may be addressed using the STOP method. A progression of trays may also be created, with one being a scene of life before using the STOP method, and the next after having used this. The sandtray therapist may also simply use this visualization prior to the creation of any tray(s).

TRADITIONAL GESTALT TECHNIQUES

In addition to the empty chair technique noted above, there are multiple other classic Gestalt techniques, many of which focus on here-and-now awareness, as well as acknowledgment of the mind, body, and emotional connection. Perls (1969) said: "Awareness, per se—by and of itself—can be curative" (p. 26). While awareness is a key, but perhaps not the key, this perspective shares the sandtray therapy focus on bringing to awareness underlying issues through the metaphor of the creative process.

As part of the sandtray creation process, a greater focus can be put on awareness. The therapist can simply ask: "What are you aware of right now?" or "What is (this miniature figure) aware of right now?" The client can also be asked to repeat or reenact a behavior, such as when clients are holding tight to or caressing a miniature, this can be brought to their attention and they can be asked to continue this action. Awareness can also be focused on another person, whether in the context of conjoint or individual therapy. Is it possible for a client—or in the case of sandtray therapy, a miniature figure—to 'become' another person? Awareness interventions can also involve self-dialogue (directly to or between figures), enactment activities, or dream work. Some other Gestalt techniques that can be used in sandtray therapy include: The *hot seat*, where a miniature is put in a place of intense focus; *mirroring*, where the therapist takes on the role of the client or the client's miniature(s), either imitating the client/miniature or providing alternative emotional or behavioral responses; suggesting *"May I feed you a sentence"*—which can be directed directly to the client or a miniature—which involves the therapist proposing a perspective or reaction to the process, and the client testing out its fit in the here-and-now moment; and encouraging clients (and again, the miniature(s)) to *stay with this feeling*, used when the client refers to a mood that is undesirable, but also engages in avoidance or denial.

SCALING QUESTIONS

Another adaption for the sandtray therapy process is the use of scaling questions. Scaling questions are commonly used in therapy across many theoretical orientations, and call for a verbal response. They can be effective in determining client self-perception and therapeutic progress. However, some clients may have challenges in coming up with a rating number, or may have a cognitive view of themselves that may not match their intrapsychic or interpersonal reality.

For example, the client may be prompted: "Some people rate their level of depression using a scale from 1 to 10. You might be able to come up with a number, but I am wondering if you could make a sandtray that would depict how depressed you feel today."

Another example would be to assess how far clients see themselves as having come in the therapy journey: "I'd be interested in your assessment of how far we've come in therapy. One way to do this is rate it on a scale—with 10 being the solution you've been looking for, and 1 being the place you were at when you came in for counseling. Instead of this, I'm wondering if you could make a sandtray that depicts where you see yourself today."

An adaption of this could be: "Today, I'd like to ask you to do two sand trays. The first would be a scene of how you were when you first came in for counseling, and the second would be a scene of where you see yourself now." This could be further adapted by showing the client a picture taken of an earlier sandtray: "This is a picture of one of the trays you did when you first came in for counseling. It seems like you've come a long way. Looking at this, I wonder if you could make a tray that shows where you feel you're at today."

Another way scaling questions are used in therapy is to ask clients to rate how others might perceive their current functioning. This can be nicely adapted to the sandtray, by asking clients to create trays instead. For example: "If your partner/employer/friend was here, and I asked them to make a tray about you, I wonder what that would look like. It might be tough to do this, but please make the tray you think they'd make."

IDENTIFYING/PROCESSING COGNITIVE DISTORTIONS

Cognitive therapy (CT) is frequently used with a wide variety of presenting issues. Essentially, CT looks to adjust information processing as a basis for cognitive change, with the hope of modifying dysfunctional interpretations that affect behavioral, emotional, and cognitive responses (Beck & Weishaar, 2005). A primary strategy is the identification and modification of cognitive distortions. These distortions can be identified and modified though the sandtray therapy process. The following are some of CT's primary identified cognitive distortions (Beck & Weishaar, 2005), and how they might be addressed in sandtray therapy.

Arbitrary inference is defined as "drawing a specific conclusion without supporting evidence or even in the face of contradictory evidence" (p. 247). This might emerge in the sandtray with a scene of the father who feels like a parental failure because he missed his son's soccer game when he needed to work an overtime shift: "I understand that attending this game meant a lot to you, and both you and your son were disappointed. If you made a sandtray about your being a father, however, I expect that this scene would take up a very small portion of the tray. I wonder if you could make a tray about how you feel about being a father, and some of the things you've been able to do with your son."

Selective abstraction is defined as "conceptualizing a situation on the basis of a detail taken out of context, ignoring other information" (p. 247). This might emerge in the sandtray with the client who becomes suspicious of a colleague who gets a promotion because her office location is closer to the supervisor's: "It must be frustrating not to get this promotion that you were expecting. It's hard to say how much office location played in the decision, but since you don't have control over that, I wonder if you could make a tray about several things you could change in your work that could help for the next promotion cycle." This could help clients focus on what they do have control over, as well as explore other possibilities for the missed opportunity.

Overgeneralization is defined as "abstracting a general rule from one or a few isolated incidents and applying it too broadly and to unrelated situations" (p. 247). This might emerge with the man who has a disappointing date with a woman and paints all women negatively: "It does sound like that date did not go as you wanted it to. You've

> Often the hands know how to solve a riddle with which the intellect has wrestled in vain (Jung, 1971, p. 294).

got some bad feelings about this woman, but I wonder if all women are really like that. Could you do a sandtray with two sides—on one side, make a scene about how you feel about this woman you dated, and on the other side, make a scene about the kind of woman you would really like to build a relationship with."

Magnification and minimization is defined as "seeing something as far more significant or less significant than it actually is" (p. 247). This might emerge for the woman who is catastrophizing that her presentation was a failure because she had a runny nose: "I'm not going to try to talk you out of how you're feeling, but I would like to look at something else. Since you were selected to make this presentation, could you do a sandtray about how you wish it had gone? And, what did people miss out on because of your runny nose?"

Personalization is defined as "attributing external events to oneself without evidence supporting a causal connection" (p. 247). This might emerge for the graduate student whose greeting to a professor in a crowded and noisy room receives no response, means that the professor was offended, which will negatively affect grades: "It could be that the professor was ignoring you, or perhaps a number of other things. If we divide the sandtray into eight small sections, each representing why the professor didn't respond—one of which is that you offended him—could you fill in the other spaces with other possibilities?"

Dichotomous thinking is defined as "categorizing experiences in one or two extremes; for example, as complete success or failure" (p. 247). This might emerge with the client who has run for an organization's elected position and lost, and now feels like a professional failure: "It is discouraging to lose—I wouldn't even want to try to convince you otherwise. We can focus on why this happened if you'd like, but not for right now. For now, I wonder if you could do a sandtray about your job and the things you like about it." Our expectation is that someone able to run for an elected position is already firmly established in a job, and the needed training and qualifications to get there. This is where this client needs to focus, before considering the negative circumstance.

DIALECTICAL BEHAVIOR THERAPY (DBT)

Dialectical Behavior Therapy (DBT) is an empirically validated approach to behavior therapy that was originally developed to treat suicidal ideation and clients diagnosed with borderline personality disorder (Linehan, 1993). Fundamentally, the theoretical basis of DBT is the dialectical philosophy that two, ostensibly opposing elements can be true at the same time (Linehan). Regulating acceptance that these elements exists are as they need or are meant to be, with the concurrent truth that the status needs to change is an illustration of the process of dialectical philosophy.

There are some basic similarities between sandtray therapy and DBT that suggest that the integration of the two is an exciting possibility. Some examples: 1) Sandtray therapy is focused on the tray and the process creating a container, and DBT places emphasis on distress tolerance—which is arguably assisted and attained within the context of *temenos*; 2) As an expressive therapy, sandtray therapy looks to develop metaphorical and literal awareness and insight, and DBT has a significant focus on mindfulness; 3) Sandtray therapy seeks to create a holding environment, which is matched by DBT's focus on maintaining an egalitarian perspective; and 4) Sandtray therapy offers the opportunity for symbolization and sublimation through the creation process and the miniature figures, and DBT places emphasis on emotional regulation—which is assisted by the therapeutic distance created through this symbolic and sublimating dynamic.

Linehan and Wilks (2015) summarize the four skills modules of DBT:

1. mindfulness
2. interpersonal effectiveness
3. emotional regulation
4. distress tolerance.

They note that: "Each skills module has at least one mindfulness skill, e.g., mindfulness of others in interpersonal skills, mindfulness of current emotions in emotion regulation, and mindfulness of current thoughts in distress tolerance" (pp. 103–104). The sandtray therapy process can help with these skills, as noted in the mindfulness section above.

Additionally, sandtray therapy can assist teaching these skills through role-playing. Miniature figures can act out interpersonal effectiveness through various sandtray creation scenarios. The client can be taught emotional regulation through the counselor coaching through the miniature figures, and transferring the skills to the client's personal relational situations. Clients can also practice distress tolerance, for example, through considering how one or more miniature figures might handle stressful situations. Sandtray therapists can adapt the exercises in Linehan's (2015a) *DBT Skills Training Manual* to the sandtray process, and then send clients home with follow-up homework from Linehan's (2015b) *DBT Skills Training Handouts and Worksheets*. Obviously, therapists adapting DBT into the sandtray therapy process should have adequate training and supervised experience with DBT as well as sandtray therapy.

CONCLUSION

Sandtray therapy creates an ideal place for the *experience* of cognitive and structured techniques. For many clients, especially children, experience carries more value than an explanation. Clients may be able to practice social skills, cognitive restructuring, and exposure to anxiety-provoking material, problem solving, and so on. A simple comment from the therapist about a sandtray miniature that has experienced pain (perhaps directly representative of the client's experience, or more general) can positively impact a client. Some examples might be: "People (or animals) shouldn't be hurt like that," or "It must be lonely (or scary) for that animal, who just can't protect him/her self." Such comments can touch a client's intrapsychic pain and open the door for deeper or more direct processes.

There are multiple presenting problems and techniques that can be used that are beyond the scope of this short chapter. Sandtray therapy can be used with such situations as relapse prevention, suicide assessment and intervention, guided imagery, grief recovery, and assertiveness training. Also, we would assert that the cross-theoretical nature of sandtray therapy can be adapted to a wide variety of approaches to counseling: From psychodynamic and behavioral, to humanistic and cognitive, constructivist to systemic—and so on!

The appropriate timing of structured interventions in the sandtray is a crucial consideration. If clients have not experienced adequate therapeutic safety and processing of intrapsychic issues, becoming too directive too early can be intrusive and discounting. Gil (2006) cautions the therapist to avoid the temptation to quickly make observations, or ask questions, particularly in case of posttraumatic sandtray work. However, an opportunity for problem solving may be lost if the sandtray therapist does not take advantage of an established therapeutic rapport and the ability to adapt the sandtray process in a more direct manner.

As noted, there are a myriad of possible adaptations of structured techniques to the sandtray therapy process. Readers are encouraged to use the imagination that led to becoming sandtray therapists in the consideration of all of the possibilities.

8

Group Sandtray Therapy

Groups are so exciting. The energy group members bring is enlivening and synergistic. Groups provide multiple opportunities to build relationship and develop communication skills. They develop community. They promote vicarious learning, developing self-awareness, willingness to self-disclose, developing an ability to enter each other's worlds, and have others enter theirs.

There are several types of sandtray therapy groups: individuals working within group setting, same age groups, family groups, parent-child dyads, sibling groups, supervision groups, personal growth groups, and professional development experiences. Groups can be found in schools, agencies, private practice, in-service training experiences, and other areas.

There are a wide variety of specific group sandtray therapy interventions. Many of the techniques discussed in Chapters 7 through 9 can be adapted for use with groups. As noted multiple times in our book, one of the benefits of sandtray therapy is that it can be employed cross-theoretically and is adaptable for a wide variety of techniques. Recognizing some of the dynamics noted in this chapter, we would encourage readers to explore adaptation of many group techniques to the sandtray therapy process. In addition to exploring adaptations from our other books, *The Handbook of Group Play Therapy* (Sweeney & Homeyer, 1999) and *Group Play Therapy: A Dynamic Approach* (Sweeney, Baggerly, & Ray, 2014), we suggest exploring basic group therapy resources to adapt both classic and novel techniques to the sandtray therapy process (see, for example: Corey, Corey, & Corey, 2014; Fehr, 2017; Jacobs, Schimmel, Masson, & Harvill, 2012; Viers, 2007). Also see group sandtray therapy research in Chapter 12.

WHY DO GROUP SANDTRAY THERAPY?

Adapted from Sweeney et al. (2014), there are several benefits and rationale for using group sandtray therapy:

1. Groups tend to promote spontaneity in clients, thus increasing their level of participation in the sandtray therapy experience. The therapist's attempt to communicate permissiveness is further enhanced by group dynamics.
2. The affective life of group members is explored at several levels—intrapsychic as well as interpersonal issues—between the therapist and clients, as well as among the clients themselves.
3. Sandtray therapy groups provide opportunities for vicarious learning. Clients observe the emotional and behavioral expressions of other group members and learn coping behaviors and alternative avenues of self-expression.
4. Clients experience the opportunity for self-growth and self-exploration in group sandtray therapy. This is promoted through self-reflection/insight as they learn to evaluate and reevaluate themselves in light of peer feedback.

5. Sandtray therapy groups serve as a microcosm of society, and the therapist has the opportunity to gain substantial insight into client's everyday lives.

6. The group sandtray therapy setting may decrease the need or tendency to be repetitious and/or to retreat into fantasy play. The group sandtray therapy setting can bring clients 'stuck' in repetition or fantasy into the here and now.

7. Clients have the opportunity to 'practice' for everyday life in the group sandtray therapy process. Clients have the opportunity to develop interpersonal skills, master new behaviors, offer and receive assistance, and experiment with alternative expressions of emotions and behavior.

8. The presence of more than one client in the sandtray setting may assist in the development of the therapeutic relationship. As withdrawn or avoidant clients observe the therapist building trust with other clients, they are often drawn in.

WORKING WITH GROUPS

When developing a sandtray therapy group experience, clearly identifying the purpose of the group will guide the selection of group members. Here are a few reminders for putting a group together. Remember developmental age. If working with very young children, probably two or three is sufficient. The group experience will be more like holding concurrent sessions as young children alternate between cooperative play and individual play. They will weave back and forth between these types of play. At times it will seem like you are holding two separate sandtray therapy sessions that just happen to be occurring in the same room at the same time. With younger children, mixing genders is quite appropriate. For groups made up of older children, single-gender groups may be preferable. This removes the growing dynamics of sexual issues complicating interactions during the sessions. Family sandtray therapy groups provide the opportunity for all members of the family to be fully involved with the wide variety of developmental ages. The family sessions become truly inclusive.

SETTING UP GROUP SPACE

Ideally, an office that is set aside for group sandtray therapy is best (Sweeney et al., 2014). A room that includes typical office equipment may be a challenge, as the clients may look beyond the collection of miniature figures for materials to add to the tray(s). Recognizing the challenge in having these facilities, the group sandtray therapist must structure the room in a manner that places the focus on the tray(s) and miniature figures, minimize access to "non-sandtray" materials, and be prepared to set therapeutic limits.

The amount of space you have for doing group sandtray therapy will naturally dictate the size of the group. There must be sufficient space to allow physical movement of group members around the sandtray and to and from the collection of miniature figures. The collection of miniature figures needs to be well organized as mentioned earlier in this book. Because more people will be using the collection of miniature figures, it must be a sufficiently adequate collection. Having said this, the collection does not need to be—for example, for a group of four people—four times the size of a typical collection. The collection also does not need to have four of each item. A benefit of the group process is learning how to share and manage limited resources. However, because we also believe that the miniature figures are the client's words, symbols, and are used to develop metaphors, we also need to have a sufficient number and variety of figures so group members can express themselves.

If working with preschoolers, deep trays are more helpful to everyone concerned. Young children are quite active, continually moving the items in the sand tray as if

. . . if you and six of your colleagues can play together once weekly for a year with the collection you are offering your clients in group and you are able to express yourselves without difficulty, your collection is adequate for a group of seven children or adults, regardless of their diagnosis (De Domenico, 1999, p. 226).

doing play therapy in miniature. The sand often flies around simply as a part of the playing. In this situation it is inappropriate to set limits, as the spilling of the sand comes from normal, age-appropriate movement. Therefore, deeper trays help contain this activity removing the unneeded distraction of the accidental spilling of sand.

It is easy and relatively inexpensive to construct a group sand tray that can be put together for the group experience, and then put out of the way until needed again. Everything can be found at a home center store and no carpentry skills are needed. Ask for two six-foot-long, 1-inch by 4-inch (called 1-by-4's) pieces of wood to be cut in half. These will serve as the four sides of the sandtray. Use corner braces (found in the carpentry section of the store) to hold the four pieces of wood together, as seen in Figure 8.1. Drape a blue painter's cloth inside the wooden sides and fill with two bags of play sand. Voila! You have a three-foot-square group sand tray. This size will easily accommodate 5 to 7 people, as seen in Figure 8.2. Also available at home centers stores

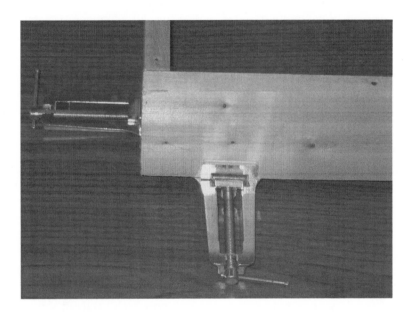

FIGURE 8.1   Corner of group sand tray

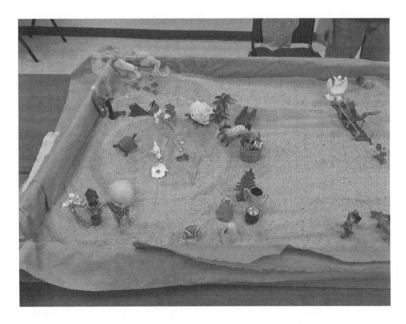

FIGURE 8.2   Group sand tray in use

are 5-gallon buckets. One bucket is large enough to hold the sand, the blue cloth, and corner brackets in these buckets until needed again. Word to the wise, be sure the sand is dry before putting in the cloth and brackets and putting on the lid.

Often the group sandtray therapist may desire to artificially and temporarily divide the group sandtray into sections. For example, this may be valuable when working with enmeshed or disengaged families or shifting from individual trays to group sand tray. This is easily done in a group sand tray by using dividers such as dowels. (Again, dowels are available at home center stores where they will cut them to your requested lengths.) In the 3-foot by 3-foot sand tray just described, dowels of about 18 inches provide several uses. For example, use the dowels to divide the tray into four quadrants for a family of four. Family members initially have their own section in which to work, while still participating within the larger family tray. At some appropriate time in the therapeutic process, the dividers can be reconfigured to have space for a parent subsystem and another for the children subsystem. The family can then work on realigning these subsystems, which are often in disarray because of a number of systemic issues. Finally, all dividers may be removed for the family to collectively create together in the sand tray.

WORKING WITH INDIVIDUALS IN A GROUP SETTING

Group sandplay is an intervention designed specifically to utilize both parallel and joint play in a therapeutic environment that encourages safety, a sense of belonging, and exploration of self in relationship to others. (Kestly, 2001, pp. 261–262)

One format for group counseling is to have individuals work in their own individual sand trays in a group setting. This is clearly a form of parallel play. The plan can be to use this format for the entire group experience. Or, it might be to shift the individuals in the group to a group sandtray at an appropriate time in the process. Teresa Kestly (2001, 2010) has written and taught a group process of individual work within a group, which she calls *sandtray friendship groups*. Kestly recommends groups of two to six or more. Groups with higher numbers of children would need more than one group facilitator. When ready to shift from the individual trays to the large communal tray, Kestly suggests that the large group tray be on the floor and 4- to 5-feet square, or in diameter, if working with a large group of children. She recommends 10 to 12 weekly sessions of about one hour in length. Younger children (kindergarten and first grade) may find 45 minutes adequate. The sessions begin with building time with a 5-minute warning when the allotted building time is about completed. The remaining 15 to 20 minutes is used for sharing the stories of their trays. She reminds us that young children will find it difficult to stay quiet while others are telling their tray stories. The therapist, being sensitive to this age-appropriate situation, can allow young children to play quietly in their trays while others are talking. The therapist will need to use therapeutic prompts to assist children in telling their stories and keep other children attentive and nonintrusive. In the research chapter you can read studies based in part on her protocol.

Gisela De Domenico (1999) discussed the behavior of children working individually in a group sandtray setting. She indicates that as group members look at each other's trays, they show respect for the other group members' worlds. The children like to 'visit' each other's worlds, commenting on each other's ingenuity of building in the tray. They also helped solve each other's building dilemmas. They are eager to hear other's stories. As a group experience will facilitate, children are able to work out on their own a new way to interact with each other.

Applying Yalom's (2005) therapeutic factors, group members note the similarities in their trays. This universality is a key dynamic—both in miniatures and meaning. As group members visit each other's trays, a certain amount of copying or 'contamination' will occur from one builder to another. For example, in one fifth-grade boys group, one boy placed a small blue foam container or box (it once held fruit) into the sand and filled it with water. It subsequently appeared in all the other boys' trays. The universality of learning that one is not alone occurs in group sandtray therapy just as in other group experiences. This dynamic counters the elements of secrecy and isolation. It removes the 'being different' feeling that members bring into a group experience. The ability to develop insight into others' experiences that may be alike or very different than one's own also occurs. This toleration of different viewpoints is critical for the development of empathy and respect of others.

In order to shift from advanced individual work to a communal sand tray requires more trust, patience, faith, interest in one another, and tolerance of other's attitudes and behaviors (De Domenico, 1999). A group ego is developed and the members' understanding of the impact of their own action on others increases.

GROUP SANDTRAY SUPERVISION

We have also used this format of individual trays in the group format in the context of group supervision. Carnes-Holt, Meany-Walen and Felton (2014) write that a "sandtray exercise in clinical supervision can be intentionally utilized for purposes such as examining cases, improving conceptualization skills, increasing self-awareness, and exploring relationship dynamics" (p. 502–503). As counselor educators and supervisors, we have both found the use of the sand tray to be a valuable tool in the clinical supervision process.

Anekstein, Hoskins, Astramovich, Garner and Terry (2014) proposed the following model of group sandtray supervision:

1. Introduce supervisees to the sand trays and the available tools.
2. Ask the supervisees to close their eyes for a brief relaxation exercise of concentrating on their breathing.
3. Give supervisees the Bernard's (1979) Discrimination Model-based directive to reflect on specific clients with whom they are working and then reflect on

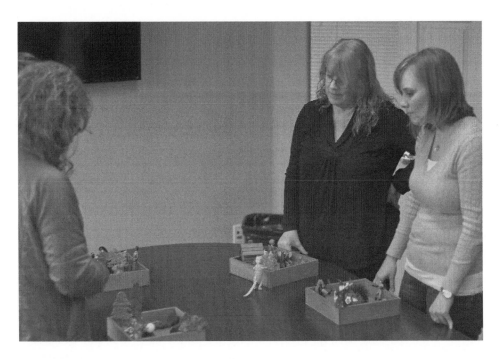

FIGURE 8.3   Group sandtray supervision

the three foci of supervision (intervention, conceptualization, and personalization) of Bernard's Discrimination Model. Encourage them to use one, two, or all three components. Have supervisees use the sandtray to illustrate how they have been working with their clients.

4. Process the sandtrays of the supervisees in the following steps:
    a. observe while the supervisees are creating the sand trays;
    b. ask the supervisees to name the theme of the sand trays;
    c. ask the supervisees which foci (intervention, conceptualization, or personalization) are being illustrated;
    d. ask supervisees to discuss the sandtray worlds and process from general to specific;
    e. invite the supervisees to give voices to the figurines;
    f. ask supervisees which foci of supervision (intervention, conceptualization, or personalization) identified by Bernard's (1979) Discrimination Model they now see in their sandtrays after discussing them; and
    g. invite the supervisees to make any changes and rename the themes of the sandtrays.
5. Ask the supervisees for any additional feedback.
6. Give the supervisees the option to photograph the sandtray.
7. Document the session and clean up materials.
                    (Anekstein, Hoskins, Astramovich, Garner and Terry, 2014, p. 127)

Our experience with group sandtray in the supervision process is that supervisees gain both clinical insight and personal confidence as growing therapists. Individual trays in the group supervison process are valuable, and a group tray leads to increased cohesion of the supervision group.

GROUP PHASES

De Domenico (1999) identified phases of group sandtray therapy. These are similar to the stages of the general understanding of other group processes and stages. The initial, or early phase, finds that members are tense, apprehensive, and anxious. They are territorial and possessive. We know this is the time when group members are trying to find out how they fit in, if it is safe to share, and what are the group rules that they need to follow. The role of the therapist is that of a witness, to reflect the process, but not to interpret. As sharing occurs, safety grows, resulting in more genuine responses. Empathy and curiosity increases. Group members learn how to claim their own space and their contribution to the trays and group process. The group members learn of their own unique impact on the world as they explore concepts of personal and social responsibility. For those groups where all members are working within the same tray, this stage is marked by each person working in their own space. No relationship between the creations exists. It is as if each group member does their own building without paying any attention to the building of others.

As the process continues, group cohesion begins to take shape. The second stage is marked by the group members' issues surrounding rejection, exclusion, inclusion, and need for support. As the sense of belonging increases, the member becomes more aware of the group vision for the world being created. As group acceptance increases, the involvement in the development of group ideas increases. This will show in the tray as individuals are still creating in their own area of the tray. However, the group members begin discussing what they each are creating and will begin to add secondary items to the tray, to in some artificial way bridge or connect the individual creations. If the group tells the story of the group tray, the story will be linked in some way, but in a very disjointed way. We will also see that personal issues will show themselves in the sandtray before the group member is prepared to be aware of it or can talk about it.

Stage 3 is marked by individuals selecting miniature figures, but then discussing the emerging story with group members before or during placement in the sand tray. As the story unfolds, more figures are added to increase cohesiveness in the story. This is what is typically labeled as the working stage. Directed prompts can be valuable at this stage to focus the group on specific therapeutic issues.

Stage 4 is identified when group members have a sense of a self-created community. It is identified as cooperation and the development of relationships. Group members display their excitement regarding the synergy of their group world. The group members' building will now be marked with some discussion as they select their miniatures. The cohesion of the miniature figures and stories greatly increases.

> You will see a history of human civilization emerge before your eyes (De Domenico, 1999, p. 227).

Finally, Stage 5 is identified by the integrated story. The group members will now discuss what they plan to build in the tray before the selection of miniatures. The tray is created with the story in mind and there may continue to be changes and modifications of the story. The creation is clearly community-based and relational.

As we teach sandtray therapy courses, workshops, and seminars, we both take note of observing these stages throughout the participants group work. In graduate-school course work it is noted students naturally progress through these stages across the semester as they develop group cohesiveness. Even in 1-day trainings, the stages are noted. Groups of participants who know each other (for example, several counselors from the same agency) jump right in to Stage 4 or 5, having previously established safety and cohesion. Meanwhile, other groups made up of those who have no previous relationship begin with trays easily identified in Stage 1. It is an interesting and validating phenomenon.

THEORETICAL APPROACHES TO GROUP SANDTRAY THERAPY

There are many theoretical approaches to play therapy and group play therapy, and thus many approaches to group sandtray therapy. Four of these are briefly discussed.

From the *person-centered approach*, Landreth and Sweeney (1999) assert that child-centered group play therapy

> is based on an abiding trust in the group's ability to develop its own potential through its movement in a positive and constructive direction . . . This has significant implications for children, who are so often evaluated and so rarely given choices. The facilitator of a children's group should be very intentional to help each child to feel safe enough to grow (or not to grow) and make choices. (p. 44)

In the person-centered group sandtray therapy process, therapists provide minimal structure and direction—focusing on the facilitation and promotion of autonomy to group members. Rogers (1951) hypothesized that the self grows and changes as a result of continuing interaction with the phenomenal field. In the person-centered group sandtray process, the group and the sand tray become the phenomenal field. The therapist's responsibility is thus to keep the focus on these dynamics.

Adlerian group sandtray therapists consider group dynamics within the context of the essential phases of individual psychology. Kottman (1999) suggests: "In some ways, a group approach is ideal for working with children using Adlerian play therapy—especially during the second (exploring the lifestyle), third (helping the child gain insight into the lifestyle), and fourth (reorientation/reeducation) phases" (p. 66). Since the Adlerian perspective places emphasis on the social stimuli that motivate behavior, as well the search for such elements as mastery, superiority, social interest (which focuses a person's lifestyle)—the group sandtray therapist challenges client beliefs and goals within the context of these dynamics emerging in the sandtray creations. A variety of interventions are used, while working through the four standard phases of Adlerian therapy. It is active process, as Sonstegard (1998) states: "In Adlerian group work, learning follows from action; group participation is the necessary action for therapeutic effects" (p. 221).

Jungian group sandtray therapy looks to the group as a container for both group members and the group itself. Bertoia (1999) summarizes

> The general format in all Jungian group play therapy is to enter the work at a conscious level using clear rational language in the here-and-now. Within the session work deepens into the nonrational or metaphoric language of the unconscious. The sessions conclude by returning to external reality and firmly anchoring children in the present. (p. 93)

Although the majority of Jungian work in the sand tray is done with individuals, there can be great power in the group process. It is possible that the group can tap into deeper levels of the psyche, which can then promote a deeper expression of archetypal energy. Jung himself somewhat distrusted groups, but Bertoia posits that the interface between group members "establishes an interconnected field" and the group "collective can explore its behaviors and attitudes, and so become more conscious and adaptive as psyche directs" (p. 92). Jungian sandtray groups require the therapist to be directive, negotiating between the conscious and unconscious of group members and the group as a whole.

Gestalt group sandtray therapy focuses on contact and awareness, as Oaklander (1999) states

> The group is an ideal setting for children to enhance their contact skills . . . It is natural for children, as well as an important developmental task, to seek out other children . . . One's process in a group may be much different in a one-to-one therapy setting. When the behavior becomes foreground, we can examine it from all sides, play with it, change it. (pp. 166–167)

Since Gestalt therapy is keenly focused on experience, the group can be a supportive foundation for experience. The sandtray group promotes greater awareness of the here-and-now, amplified by the use of miniature figures in the sandtray creation. The sandtray creations and fellow group members amplify drama, and thus participation. The contact that is crucial in Gestalt therapy can be initially made through the miniature figures and the tray, and then bridged to group members. Additionally, the group sandtray process can facilitate bringing the "past into the now," which is a Gestalt priority.

GROUP SANDTRAY THERAPY TECHNIQUES

As noted, a wide variety of sandtray therapy techniques and group therapy techniques can be adapted for use in group sandtray therapy. These may vary according to theoretical approach as well as preferred technical application. They may also vary according to the use of individual trays in the group setting or a group communal tray.

In addition to adapting techniques from other chapters in this book, some other group sandtray techniques include

■ Psychodrama interventions, including using miniatures in interviews, soliloquy, role playing, and mirroring.

- Action interventions, such as empty chair, dialogue creation and re-creation, and rehearsal techniques.
- Psychodynamic interventions, including dream creations/analysis with miniature figures, exploring resistance and transference.
- CBT/REBT/SFBT interventions, including using miniature figures to engage in cognitive restructuring, challenging cognitive distortions, disputing faulty beliefs, miracle question, scaling, and motivational interviewing.
- Adaptions of creative arts interventions, including sandtray adaptions of: puppet play, collage, storytelling, finger-painting (with or without miniatures), self-portrait.

GROUP SANDTRAY THERAPY CASE

A favorite use of group sandtray therapy for both of us as counselor educators is to do group work in the classroom. We have students create trays, with the following prompt: "Make a scene in the sand that shows how you feel about being in graduate school." The students themselves are typically surprised at both how enjoyable and how powerful the experience of creating the scene is for them. In the processing of the scenes, students are able to quickly get in touch with their own issues, and understand, firsthand, the power this medium has for clients.

The following is an example of a graduate student's tray, accompanied by a verbatim written summary by the student (see Figure 8.4).

I selected an octopus at first glance because of the many roles I have played throughout my graduate experience. Often times I was unsure of what one 'tentacle' was doing at any one time. I have felt a frustrating inability to give fully to any one tentacle, all being important for various reasons. I then chose miniatures that expressed each of these priorities.

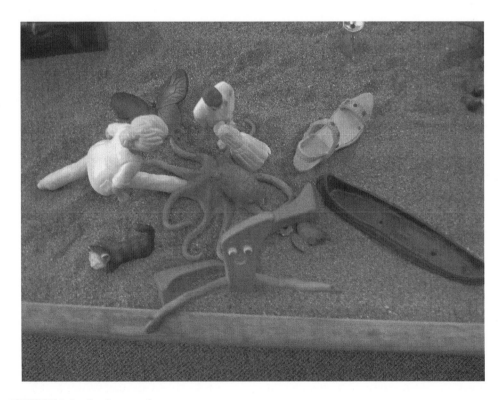

FIGURE 8.4   Graduate student tray

I found a bride and groom that appeared happy. My role as a wife is a passion and a delight in my life. However, I leaned the bride into the groom, displaying the reality that at times I have maybe leaned more into my husband than he has into me. I know he has sacrificed a lot while I have been in school, and at times I felt like I might need to quit in order to maintain my 'part' in the relationship.

I picked a large Gumby™, that displayed my feelings of being molded, shaped, bendable, and even at times, too flexible, as I soaked in the learning experiences. Gumby also has a confused look on his face—which I think I have worn often throughout my experience! I chose a professional woman doctor to portray my full-time job [counseling] at a large church. She appeared sure of herself and someone that others looked to for help . . . I think Gumby and the Doctor were of equal size.

I chose a woman's high-heel [shoe], revealing the side of me that desires to remain playful and feminine in a masculine world. Being in academia, this has been a hard one to hold tight to over the years. I chose a chicken, representing the side of me that is afraid to move forward. I chose a boat, representing the journey I have been on with God and the places of rest and hardship I have faced thus far and throughout grad school. My relationship with God has kept me sane! I also chose a butterfly, which I believe reflects my deepest desire to be transformed . . . I believe this graduate process is part of that process.

This is quite a powerful and insightful experience, particularly considering that this tray was done as part of a group tray experience and in a classroom setting. Despite the typically non-therapeutic conditions, sandtray therapy has a way of reaching quite deep in a group setting.

9

Sandtray Therapy with Couples and Families

In the same way that our definition of sandtray therapy calls for the process to be facilitated by a trained sandtray therapist, sandtray work with couples and families calls for the therapist to have adequate training in both sandtray therapy and couple/family therapy dynamics. It is important to have adequate training in relational dynamics, communication skills, family systems, human development, and couple and family treatment models.

This training cannot be emphasized enough. In their study of family therapists who either included or excluded children from the family therapy process, Korner and Brown (1990) found that family therapists who had received specialized training with children or who felt that their training with children was adequate were those who were more likely to include children in the therapy process. Not a surprise! It is clear—family therapists who want to truly be inclusive and systemic therapists, need child therapy training—and in our opinion, sandtray therapy training!

There are many exciting prospects in the use of sandtray therapy with couples and families. In addition to the opportunities to apply traditional and novel couple and family therapy interventions within the context of the sandtray process, the discovery of communication patterns that contribute to the presenting issues becomes easier for both the therapist and clients.

Couples and family therapy can be challenging for all mental health professionals, including the sandtray therapist. It is not unusual to find one or more members of a couple or family in the therapy process reluctant to actively participate in the therapeutic process. The presenting issues are often complex and entrenched—as a result, many couples and families delay seeking treatment until a crisis develops. By then, patterns of communication and metacommunication can be difficult to assess and process (Sweeney, 2002). Additionally, when family members are unwilling or unable to verbally express themselves in their daily relationship and during the counseling process, a nonverbal means of expression such as sandtray therapy is helpful.

Family therapists and play therapists share a noble trait: They are by far the most creative and dynamic therapists in existence (Gil, 1994, p. 34).

As with individual clients, sandtray therapy allows family members (in individual or conjoint trays) the opportunity to create 'world' pictures in the sand tray, giving the counselor, and perhaps more importantly, family members, the opportunity to view relationship and communication dynamics. What family members do or do not contribute to the process is frequently a reflection of the investment that they have in the couple or family relationships. The frequent 'dance' that individual family members and couples do to avoid core issues emerges, creating an opportunity for a new waltz to begin. Triangles and the related emotional processes can be identified and resolved.

Sweeney and Rocha (2000) assert that family therapy must address the "lowest developmental denominator" (p. 36). This means including children and adolescents along with the adults. Few would deny the contribution that children make to the functioning or dysfunction of a family system, yet they are frequently excluded from the family therapy process. Sandtray therapy is inclusive, "levels the playing field between the developmental levels of family members" and provides a metaphorical blueprint of family alliances, intergenerational patterns, and stages of personality development (Sweeney & Rocha, 2000, p. 36).

Family-of-origin issues are revealed through the metaphorical process of sandtray therapy. It is the responsibility of the therapist to consider these issues with each member of the couple or family, as they contribute a great deal to the current system dynamics. So often, clients are unaware of or refuse to recognize the impact of family-of-origin issues on the presenting problem. The sandtray therapy process creates a safe and effective forum for both discovery and change.

Additionally, partners and family members bring various personality traits and communication styles into their daily relational functioning. Since frequent treatment goals of couple and family therapy include cooperation and negotiation, there is substantial benefit in fostering mutual understanding of personality and communication issues.

A variety of schools of family therapy, including strategic, systemic, experiential, and behavioral, have traditions that encourage active engagement of all-aged family members in the therapy process (Chasin, 1989). Family sculpting (Papp, Silverstein, & Carter, 1973) and structural therapy's enactment (Minuchin, 1974) are examples of such activity. The inclusion of all family members, particularly children, in family therapy provides the sandtray therapist the opportunity to observe patterns of communication, roles, coalitions, and triangles rather than making assumptions based on the self-report of one partner or a few individual family members. This helps the therapist view the complexity of interactions within the family gestalt and to observe how family dynamics are impacted by individual development and family life cycle needs. We believe if the whole family is to be treated therapeutically, the whole family should be included, which can more readily occur in sandtray therapy.

The interactional sequence described by Guerin, Fay, Burden and Kautto (1987) becomes particularly clear in the sandtray therapy process. Conflictual marriages are described as typically involving a *pursuit* and *distancing* pattern; this pattern may be evident to the couple or counselor at some level, and it is further identified in the sand tray. Identification of this reciprocal pattern is crucial to the resolution of couple conflict, so that new relationship and communication skills can be taught. Sandtray therapy, therefore, can be used as both an evaluatory and training tool in treatment.

An additional benefit to sandtray therapy with couples and families is that it naturally removes the focus off of any one partner or family member. Family therapists should always be aware of the *identified patient*, and should always work to remove this focus. Sandtray therapy, with its expressive and projective nature, facilitates the de-emphasis on the identified patient.

Some couples are willing and able to process their issues on a verbal level, and they should not be forced into using sandtray therapy in the counseling office. However, even these couples may be consciously or unconsciously denying an important concern that may emerge in the sandtray therapy process.

SANDTRAY INTERVENTIONS WITH COUPLES AND FAMILIES

In couples work, Fishbane (2013) talks about encouraging couples to see multiple realities. This can be a challenge. Is it possible to use miniature figures to explore each other's realities in the tray—rather than attempt to identify them at a cognitive level in real life? In describing her couple work, Fishbane writes: "I normalize their reactivity, which de-shames it for the couple. At the same time, I offer the possibility that they can transcend their automatic tendency to become reactive" (p. 131). We would suggest that since couples are so often reactive towards each other, this dynamic is decreased by using the miniature figures as a tool for discussing the shaming cycle, and exploring alternative ways for the figures to interact, before moving on to the couple themselves. This psychological distancing is core to the sandtray therapy process.

We would suggest that the sandtray therapist not take on the role of advice giver, problem solver, or referee in the initial stages of sandtray work with couples and families. The focus, as with individual sandtray therapy, should first be on intrapersonal and interpersonal discovery. This creates the safe place and avenue where communication development and conflict resolution can occur.

Introduction of the sandtray process with couples and families does not differ much from that with individual clients. Directions from the therapist can be either nondirected or directed.

While the choice depends on the therapist's preference as well as the presenting issue, we often begin the sandtray process with couples and families by having them create individual trays. You may determine that a conjoint tray is the place to start, but we have frequently experienced the presenting conflict to be quite palpable and tender, and the sensory and kinesthetic nature of sandtray therapy can be overwhelming in an initial conjoint tray.

The next step is to ask couples or family members to create trays side by side. This can be very important if there is a sense that one or both of couple partners or, one or more family members, appear to be unwilling or unable to adequately express themselves in a joint tray. The joint tray may be too threatening to do at this early stage of work; some family members may withdraw during the creation of a joint tray but be able to more fully express and create on an individual basis. As partners or family members create these individual trays, we normally discourage them from talking during the creation of the worlds. After they complete the trays, we will ask each partner or family member whether he or she is willing to share about the tray, and we encourage or coach the other partner in active listening. Interruptions are not allowed, and equal time is given to talk, even if the time is not used.

It is not unusual for members of a couple or family to feel that they have not been heard or do not have a voice in the current relational conflict. Individual trays provide them the opportunity to express self, to "talk" about pain, fears, and hopes through the creation of the tray. When the couple or family members share about their trays, they are not only sharing with the therapist, but also with their partners or family members.

If partners or family members are willing, we ask them to be the 'tour guide' for their partner or other family members. We remind clients that just as tour guides are experts and not to be interrupted, they are the experts on their own perspective and emotional lives—and will be given the chance to share their sandtray world without interruption or judgment. Thus, if necessary, the therapist should facilitate the 'tours' by preventing interruption. If family members have questions of each other's trays or explanations, they are free to ask *after* the tour guide's explanation or story.

It is crucial that all parties have the experience of feeling heard and understood. This will be a part of the post-creation process. We can use many of the same process questions that are used with individual clients. The process may of course vary according to the therapist's theoretical orientation or technical preference.

When the therapist determines it is appropriate, there can be movement toward conjoint work in the sand tray. We would not endorse a continued process of individual parallel trays. While this is often a desirable place to begin, movement toward conjoint work should be a cross-theoretical and appropriate treatment planning direction in which to move.

The creation of a tray together allows us to observe couple partners and family members as they live and relate. When first doing conjoint trays, we will introduce the process as we would with individual clients, and be generally nondirected. Our instructions are generally for the couple or family to create a scene or world in the sandtray, using as many or few miniatures as they would like. There is usually not a need to be more specific than this, with the exception of providing a prompt for those couples and families who are having a difficult time beginning the tray. An example of a general prompt may be simply to ask them to construct a scene reflecting the past weekend or holiday.

As the couple or family begins to select the miniature figures and place them in the sand, our own involvement in and reflection of the process varies, depending on our sense of the clients' relationship. At times we will make frequent reflective comments and engage in dialogue with the couple or family as they work, using the clients and the general tenor of the session as our guide. Sometimes we say very little, primarily with the intent to honor and revere the construction of the tray (which is essentially the uncovering of intrapsychic and interpersonal issues), a key element in the Jungian approach. The majority of the interaction occurs at the completion of the tray, when we begin to ask questions.

As the couples and families construct the trays, the sandtray therapist should consider the following questions, which may provide insight into the clients' relational dynamics:

1. Who initiates the construction of the sand tray world? Who ends the process?
2. What objects are considered, selected, and rejected? By whom? Are one person's suggestions or sections rejected by another person or partner?
3. Are any persons' miniatures touched or moved by someone else?
4. Does the couple or family work together to construct the tray? Are there separate worlds created in the one tray?
5. Did any family member or either partner send friendly or hostile messages? Did someone send a "you do your thing and I'll do mine" kind of message?
6. Who contributed the most? What is the percentage of space used by each person?
7. Do the couple partners or family members talk to each other during the process? Do they decide on a theme? If so, do they follow the theme?
8. Is the process structured or chaotic?

The answers to these questions may provide essential information about the clients' relationships. The degree of participation, reactivity, compartmentalization, territorialism, compliance, and rejection (the list may go on) observed during the construction of the tray are frequently a direct reflection of the clients' typical interactions.

As with individual clients, after the construction of the tray, we normally begin by asking them to title the world. It is a rare occurrence that a couple or family (at least one of the members) does not come up with a title. We will then ask the couple to tell a story about the tray. In individual sandtray therapy, we will ask clients to tell the therapist about the scene, to take us into their world. With couples and families, we usually ask them to talk with each other about the tray, to take each other into the world of the tray. This may be a challenge for the couple with communication problems, and the counselor may have to assist in this process. Following this extra step, we then ask the couple or family to tell us about the tray, to take the therapist into their world. It is important to give both partners and every family member an equal opportunity to share.

This process involves considerable intra- and interpersonal material coming out through the story, and we may look to elicit further information by asking further questions: "What about this figure here? What is she doing? It looks like these two are saying something to each other—what could they be talking about? Are you (either partner or any family member) in this picture? Is there anyone else you know in here? What's going to happen next (if it is an active scene)? What (not who) has the most power here?" A number of other questions may come up within the process, but it is helpful to keep them simple and open-ended, and to avoid questions that are intrusive or that jump to a conclusion. We are also interested in the couple or family processing the experience of building and sharing their world: "What was it like for each person?"

The couple or family sandtray process may be reflective of Allan's (1988) common stages in the sandtray therapy process with children, which we have found to be helpful in assessing the progress of sandtray therapy with couples and families. The first stage is *chaos*, in which the couple or family may 'dump' miniatures into the sand, often without any apparent deliberate selection. The chaos evident in the sand is reflective of the chaos and emotional turmoil in the couple or family life. Most marriage and family therapists are familiar with the 'dumping' of issues that couples and families do in the therapy room. The next stage of *struggle* may be evident, in which there may be overt or covert conflict, even 'battle' scenes. At the beginning of the creation of these scenes, often the two (or more) sides in the fight annihilate each other. In other words, the world depicts a no-win situation. Although the scene may reflect one side winning (e.g., a dominant partner over an unassertive, compliant partner, or a domineering parent in a rigid family system), it really is not a win–lose situation, it is a lose–lose situation. We have often found that in the early stages of sandtray therapy, with many client configurations, that no one survives these battles or accidents. With positive progress, and the process of building relationship and communication, the sandtray therapy moves to the third stage of *resolution*, where life seems to be 'getting back to normal.' There is more order and balance in the tray, miniatures are deliberately selected and carefully placed, and the couple or family members see themselves in the trays, often in helpful and egalitarian roles. This is usually a sign that therapy can be brought to an end.

As we've mentioned, we have found that it is helpful to take pictures of the completed sandtray creations. In addition to the documentation of the process, it is often helpful to conclude the therapy process with a "slide show" of the journey that has been embarked upon. Also, if a single tray cannot be fully processed in one session, the picture provides the visual stimulation for subsequent sessions to continue the process. It is also helpful to video record couple or family sandtray sessions, if the technology is available. Just as therapists learn so much from receiving supervision of their video recorded work, a couple or family can learn quite a bit about their communication process by watching themselves create trays by video. The therapist can take on the role of educator and coach as family members view themselves and others by video.

SPECIFIC COUPLES SANDTRAY INTERVENTIONS

There are a variety of ways to use sandtray therapy with couples, certainly not limited to the few suggestions we offer here.

Some common ways that we introduce sandtray therapy to couples would look as follows: "I know that the issues that have brought you here are tough to talk about. I'm not here to drag things out of you, but it would certainly help to find out more about the ways you two communicate. One way I've found success with this is through a type of couples counseling called sandtray therapy. Rather than my simply peppering you with questions, I'd like for you to create a scene in the sand using as many or as few miniatures as you'd like."

It is at this point that the process can stay nondirected or become more focused. One example of a more directed process would be as follows: "It seems like you two have been at odds and arguing for so long, it's hard to remember what life was like before things got this way. I'd like you to make two scenes in the tray, with one scene being a picture of what your common life feels like now, and in the other, what it was like before the conflict started." Each person makes the two scenes, either in their own tray divided in two sections, or in one large tray, divided in half, with each partner dividing the half into two parts.

One significant benefit to doing sandtray with couples is the opportunity to adapt traditional couple therapy techniques to the sandtray therapy process. Some of the techniques that are mentioned in Chapter 7, "Integrating Sandtray Therapy with a Variety of Approaches and Techniques," can also be used. One example would be using the solution-focused miracle question with couples. There are as many adaptations as there are techniques.

An example of adapting a specific marital therapy approach would involve John Gottman's (1994) "Four Horsemen of the Apocalypse," which includes *criticism, defensiveness, contempt*, and *stonewalling*. Gottman's research indicates the presence of these behavioral dynamics to be predictive of divorce. The four issues can certainly be discussed with couples at a verbal level. However, a deeper and more impactful process might involve the unfolding of these in the tray. The therapist can ask each partner: "Could you make a tray of the last time you experienced criticism/defensiveness/contempt/stonewalling in your relationship? Could you make a tray of the last time you criticized/acted defensive/expressed contempt/stonewalled in your relationship? Could you make a tray of how your partner might experience these?" Be aware that these are invitations to do so, and may be turned down. However, this is a way to honor clients and their pain.

Another adaption would be the employment of the Imago Relationship Therapy process of the "Couple's Dialogue" (Hendrix, 2010). While adequate training is recommended when using Imago techniques, the Couple's Dialogue basically consists of *mirroring* partner statements, *summarization*, *validation* (e.g., "that makes sense because . . ."), and *empathy* (e.g., "I would imagine that you feel . . ."). The fundamental process involves helping each partner to push himself or herself to move beyond being understood to being understanding of the experience of the other partner, as being different yet equally valid. This process can be extended to sandtray therapy, as each partner can give voice to miniature figures. Mirroring can feel awkward and shallow for many, but can be practiced through projection onto figures in the sand tray. Clients who might not otherwise be teachable and compliant can feel safety, as the therapist is coaching the miniatures as a prelude to coaching the clients.

Emotion-focused therapy (EFT) is another approach that can be adapted to work with couples. Johnson (1996, 2004) outlines EFT's model of nine steps in three stages. For the sake of simplifying this, the three stages include

1. Cycle de-escalation: identifying and de-escalating negative cycles that interrupt and maintain attachment security.
2. Restructuring interactional patterns: helping partners to shift interactional patterns and promote secure attachment.
3. Consolidation and integration: summarizing the treatment process in an empowering manner and consolidating new response patterns that promote stronger relational bonds.

These can be demonstrated and practiced in the sand tray through the figures. Johnson (1996) asserts that the therapist's role is one of *process consultant* as opposed to teacher or coach. We would suggest that there is no need to completely separate these roles. However, the very term *process consultant* resonates with our approach to sandtray therapy.

A specific EFT intervention that we like to use in family sandtray is the use of disquisitions—basically, storytelling in the couples' therapy process. Millikin and Johnson (2000) describe this:

> A disquisition is a third-person fantasy narrative, fable or story, ostensibly about someone other than the client. The story is intended to reflect and clarify the attachment drama implicit in the couple's interaction. Disquisitions follow the logic and structure of the clients' presenting problem and process in therapy. This narrative has specific relevance to clients' stuck points, but the therapist presents the story as tentative. A disquisition's fable-like quality places the couple's responses in a universal context, applicable to all who struggle with close bonds. Disquisitions are told in a safe, validating way and by their nature, these fables legitimize and validate each partner's responses. (p. 76)

Sandtray therapy is a wonderful way to employ EFT's disquisitions. The therapist is the storyteller, and the story is graphically narrated, with the background being the sand tray and the characters being the miniatures.

SPECIFIC FAMILY SANDTRAY INTERVENTIONS

As with couples, there are a myriad of possible uses of sandtray therapy with families, including the few suggested here. Once again, there are as many adapted sandtray applications as there are techniques.

We were just talking about the therapist acting as a coach, which is a role that many family therapists identify with, including Murray Bowen (1976). By taking the role of a coach, rather than expert, clients are more readily able to engage in the process of change by taking personal responsibility. As noted, it may be easier for clients to receive coaching through the sandtray miniatures, as a gradual process toward personal ownership.

One adaption of a family therapy technique to sandtray is the use of sculpting (Papp, Silverstein, & Carter, 1973). This traditionally involves providing each family member the opportunity to physically 'sculpt' the family structure through the positioning of family members according to the individual's perspective. This is often done with chairs in the therapy room, which can certainly provide a picture of the family dynamics for both the therapist and the family. Younger family members, particularly children, however, are placed at an automatic disadvantage in this process. To ask some family members to perform such a task is often an overwhelming requirement. Even when family members are able, the older family members often influence the sculpted structure, particularly when one considers the general nature of children, who are so often focused on pleasing parents and adults. This can be easily resolved through instructing the family to 'sculpt' their family members in the sandtray, using miniatures of their choice. The specific selection of miniatures is instructive, and family members often feel freer to display the family hierarchy when doing so projectively.

Another effective family sandtray intervention is the creation of a genogram using sandtray miniatures. Genograms are a wonderful "map" to family structure and dynamics (for further information on genograms, see McGoldrick, Gerson, & Petty, 2008). Therapists simply ask family members to select one or more miniatures that show their thoughts and feelings about every member of the family, including themselves (Gil, 2003). This should be done on a piece of paper, rather than using the sand tray. The therapist or the family can draw the genogram outline, using the customary squares (for males) and circles (for females), including the lines that correspond to the family relationship. Miniature figures are then selected to be placed on top of the squares and circles. For example, one client used an alcohol bottle to symbolize an alcoholic father and an angel figure for his mother. Every miniature can become a powerful symbolic message about family members.

It is the therapist's call as to how this process unfolds. We will often have family members choose figures simultaneously, as this can prevent the self-consciousness that can develop if family members are compelled to select while others are watching. After the selection, the therapist facilitates discussion of the miniatures chosen. Obviously, a great deal of insight can be gained through the processing of symbolic and metaphorical meanings of these miniatures.

This sandtray genogram can also be extended to another part of the genogram process. In traditional genograms, various line configurations and symbols are used to depict relationships (e.g., three parallel lines indicates enmeshment, a jagged line indicates conflict, etc.). With this adaptation, family members can also select miniatures to represent their perspective on the nature of family relationships. Obviously, the selection of a miniature wall would be very telling about how one family member perceives his/her relationship with another. One might find bridges, lines of precious stones or marbles, or even walls and fences used to depict relationships between family members.

Another effective adaptation of traditional family therapy would be through the structural family therapy use of *enactment*. Fundamentally, an enactment is the therapist staging an outside family conflict in the therapy setting, in order to evaluate and process a path for change (Colapinto, 2000). Through the use of sandtray therapy, the therapist and family members can get a three-dimensional and kinesthetic view of family conflicts, as scenes are displayed or acted out with miniatures in the sandtray.

A classic example of a family therapy intervention is to have family members take on a paradoxical role. Weeks and L'Abate (1982) give some instructions:

> Assume the symptom is a daughter's acting-out and taking charge in the single parent family. The daughter is told to exaggerate her taking charge of her mother. At the same time, the mother is told to assume the paradoxical role of the child. She is instructed to give up her position of authority and to be a helpless child. (p. 91)

This can be role-played with miniature figurines in the sand tray, which can facilitate what may otherwise be a challenging activity to verbally process.

A cognitive-behavioral family technique can be behavior rehearsal. While this is frequently done verbally, the demonstrative nature of sandtray therapy can further enhance the verbal coaching done by the therapist. The goal is to practice in therapy what is intended to generalize to the family's home environment. The miniature figures can be chosen by each family member to represent self, and they serve in the role of the family members for the behavior rehearsal process. This is similar to Minuchin's coaching process noted above. Dattillio (2010) suggests that behavioral rehearsal is "one of the most essential parts of the treatment sequence because it provides feedback to the therapist regarding the extent to which couples and families have understood what they have learned and can demonstrate how it should be implemented" (p. 141).

Many other family therapy techniques can be adapted, including Madanes' (1984) *pretend techniques*, Guerin's (1971, as cited in Nichols, 2013) *displacement story*—with further displacement onto the miniatures, the *rituals* of the Milan Model (Boscolo, Cecchin, Hoffman, & Penn, 1987), paradoxical techniques such as *prescribing the symptom* (Weeks & L'Abate, 1982), and the *definitional ceremonies* of narrative family therapy (White, 2007). All of these can be prescribed and then unfolded in the sandtray, using miniatures to dramatize the therapeutic dynamic. These are but a few of the many possible intervention applications.

COUPLES CASE EXAMPLE

This couples therapy case involved a male and female married couple in their mid-thirties who were having significant difficulty communicating and had considered divorce, but did not want to disrupt the lives of their children. We know that this sounds like a familiar scenario. It is interesting to note that they were unable or unwilling to acknowledge how their conflict was already causing disruption for the children.

Using a suggested scenario from above, this couple was asked to do a tray, creating two scenes—one of which included what they would like their marriage to look like and the other involving what it felt like currently. They were asked to work together in a single tray and divide the space as they saw fit.

An interesting dynamic occurred at the beginning of the process. As can be seen in Figure 9.1, there are two sections of the tray, divided by moving the sand to either side, creating what looked to be a river. The husband took the initiative and created the narrow "river," and then the wife widened the gap considerably. This was consistent with the initial presentation that she saw the problem as more significant than he did. Neither partner selected many miniatures for the scene. Their selections and brief explanations were, however, quite impactful for each other.

On the wife's side, on the top right section of the tray, was her picture of how she would like the marriage to be. She placed a bride and groom miniature, commenting about how happy they were when they got married. Next to them, she placed an old man and woman holding hands. She said that she had always hoped they would grow old together, and still hoped they could. She was teary-eyed as she shared this, which in turn brought tears to her husband's eyes.

She separated her two scenes with miniature traffic and warning signs, including a barrel of explosives. While their relationship was explosive at times, the miniature in this row that was most meaningful was a railroad crossing bar, which she deliberately

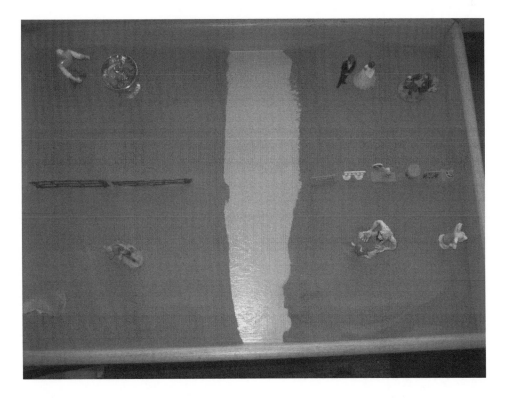

FIGURE 9.1 Couple's tray

placed upward, signifying for her that she saw hope for reconnecting. This was an interesting contrast to her having initially widened the gap between her sections and her husband's.

On the other side, which was the picture of how she saw their relationship currently, she placed Piglet (from *Winnie the Pooh*©), facing the side of the tray and turned away from everything else in the tray. She stated that this represented how small and insignificant she felt in the relationship. To represent her husband, she selected a physician figure (representing her husband's job in the health industry), facing away from Piglet, and also placed the mythical figure Gollum (from *The Lord of the Rings*©). For readers who have seen the film, you will recall him constantly saying (about the ring): "My precious." The wife, still crying, stated that she saw her husband as viewing his professional life as "precious," as opposed to her.

On the husband's side of the tray, representing how he would like the marriage to be, he placed a strong handsome male figure, reaching out to a gold chalice filled with gold nuggets. He stated that when they got married, he viewed her as valuable and precious (the chalice and gold nuggets), and that he sought after her (the outstretched arms)— and would like to regain this feeling. He stated that he had already thought of the word *precious*, which is why he responded emotionally to what his wife had shared. Needless to say, the wife was very impacted by this.

On the other side, the husband selected a translucent (almost clear) figure, which he said represented how invisible he felt in the relationship. He also placed his figure facing away from everything else in the tray. He also selected a mother and daughter, stating that he felt that his wife and daughter had built a life apart from him.

These relational dynamics were evident to the therapist, but had not been considered or explored by each partner. The most valuable aspect of this sandtray therapy experience was for each partner to hear and see the other's pain—and the other's hope for change. Whereas these dynamics and insight could certainly have been discussed at a verbal level, we would suggest that the emotional depth reached in this session would be difficult if not impossible to reach in a session limited to verbalization. In part, this is due to the visual input going directly to the right, emotional part of the brain, rather than verbal processes going only to the left side of the brain, more focused on linear, sequential, rational thought processes.

SIBLINGS CASE EXAMPLE

We have both done sandtray therapy work with children coming to counseling because of the challenge of responding to a parental divorce. The therapist can divide the tray in half or ask the client to, and give the following prompt: "On one side, build what your world was like before the divorce. On the other side, build what your world is like now." The following picture is a re-creation of a sandtray done with Daniel involving two young girls (ages 6 and 8), whose parents were divorcing. The parents were expected to also attend the session so no play therapy materials were available. When the girls showed up they were given the opportunity to make a sandtray, with the above prompt.

It may not be clear in the picture (see Figure 9.2), but the older girl chose to divide the tray in half using tombstones—certainly a vivid depiction of the death of their parents' marriage. On the left side of the tray, there is a couple, with the female figure leaning toward the male figure. They described this as how their parents were always arguing, and how their mother was particularly aggressive with her words. There are two girl figures in the lower portion of the left half, faced away from the adults and with their faces against the side of the tray. This depicted the girls' need to hide from their parents when they were fighting.

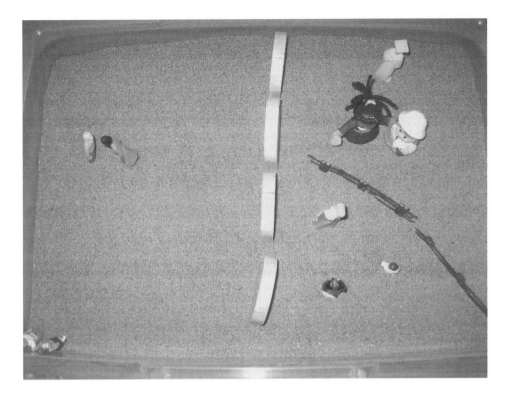

FIGURE 9.2   Sibling-children of divorce tray

On the right side of the tray, the scene was divided in half with fences. The top half was their description of living with their mother (joint physical custody at that time). They chose a female figure in academic regalia, depicting their mother's decision to go to school. They stated that their mother was going to school and dating already, and didn't have time for the girls. The two figures they selected for themselves in this section of the tray were facing away from their mother. On the bottom half of this side, the girls are facing their father (who was more relational). However, they selected the judge figure for their father, and did not discuss this selection. With the custody issue unresolved at this point, it could have represented their awareness of the judge's power in this process.

This demonstrates the vivid manner in which the sandtray process allowed the girls to access their emotions and symbols in a profoundly communicative way in the sand tray. This not only facilitated their work, but assisted the therapist obtaining information which became helpful in working with the parents during this transitional time of divorce.

CONCLUSION

The challenges of couple and family conflicts are often easier to express, observe, and process through sandtray therapy. Like any other therapeutic approach or technique, however, sandtray does not provide all of the answers. Although the primary issues related to couple and family conflict (e.g., communication, money, sex, parenting) seem to remain stable, the challenges facing families in crisis may be getting more complex. Verbalizing intrapsychic and interpersonal pain is never easy. Sandtray therapy may be one tool that provides couples and families with a safe place—a *level playing field*, if you will—in which to 'talk' about issues of great import.

Sandtray therapy reaches couples and families in unrecognized and unrealized realms. Couples and families often focus on conflict and weakness. Their possible resistance to a strength-based systemic approach can be coopted through the sandtray therapist focusing on the strengths of sandtray miniatures. Systems that resist complementarity—harmony in the meshing of roles—can see this modeled in the sand tray. Systems that have difficulty understanding differentiation can recognize its illustration in the sand tray and miniatures. Multigenerational patterns can also be illustrated through the sandtray process. Structural family therapy roles—such as blamer, placater, distractor—are more readily identified through the therapeutic distance of using miniatures to identify these roles. Hidden coalitions and subsystems are uncovered and addressed. Sandtray has great power with systems!

As with individual sandtray therapy, use of this expressive intervention may be used on a regular or intermittent basis. It has been our experience, however, that more information about communication and systemic issues can emerge from a single sandtray experience than in multiple sessions limited to verbal interaction. It is not uncommon for the great deal of intra- and interpersonal material emerging from a single sandtray experience resulting in the next several therapy sessions focusing on processing the tray(s).

As a reminder, it's our opinion that successful therapy with couples and families involves the therapist being a facilitator rather than a director of the process. Sandtray therapy naturally lends itself to this facilitation. As with sandtray therapy with any population, be encouraged to keep your focus on the process as opposed to the product.

10

Sandtray Therapy and Trauma

As with other expressive and projective interventions, sandtray therapy provides a unique and effective intervention for clients who have experienced trauma. The therapeutic distance, which is automatically provided as clients' project intrapsychic and interpersonal issues of pain and chaos into the sand tray, is an invaluable tool when doing trauma work. There are both psychological and neurobiological benefits in the use of sandtray therapy as an intervention with clients of all ages dealing with the aftermath of a trauma event(s). This chapter will comment on trauma interventions, but is more of a brief rationale for the use of sandtray therapy with traumatized clients.

To begin, an initial consideration is the fundamental sensory nature of trauma. All trauma has a sensory element to it, if not pervasive sensory overload. From the victim of a car accident to combat trauma to physical or sexual abuse, there is a significant impact on the senses of the traumatized client. Additionally, as one considers the diagnostic criteria for posttraumatic stress disorder (PTSD) in the DSM-5 (American Psychiatric Association, 2013), there is a significant focus on sensory elements: re-experiencing, avoidance, negative cognitions and mood, and arousal. The DSM-5 now includes a category for PTSD for children under six years old—however, this is not the focus of this chapter or book, and does not change our approach to sandtray therapy. Because of the significant sensory element of trauma and the DSM-5 criteria, a therapeutic response to trauma should also have a significant sensory element to it. Sandtray therapy is a natural fit.

> Badenoch writing about a client's work, "She either leaves her left hand in the sand to maintain her emerging internal balance, or holds onto one of the pieces, telling me she feels soothing energy moving up her arms and into her chest" (2008, p. 236).

BENEFITS OF SANDTRAY THERAPY FOR TRAUMATIZED CLIENTS

We have already articulated for the benefit and rationale of sandtray therapy for clients presenting with a variety of presenting problems. Issues of trauma, while particularly wounding, fit into the rationale discussed in Chapter 2. Expanding on this, Schaefer (1994) suggested several related properties that provide the sense of therapeutic distance and often resultant safety that traumatized clients can experience in sandtray therapy:

1. *Symbolization*: Clients can use a miniature to represent an abuser or victimizing situation. For example, it can be much safer for a client to select a predatory animal to represent an abuser. A client might select a jail or building with barred windows to represent being held captive, whether the presenting issue involves actual abduction or the feeling of inescapability.

2. *'As if' quality*: Clients can use the pretend quality to act out events as if they are not real life. For the victim or witness of domestic violence, for example, it is challenging enough to process this trauma verbally. In sandtray therapy, clients can manage the unmanageable, controlling in the *as if* element of the

sandtray therapy that which could not be controlled in the midst of the traumatizing situation.

3. *Projection*: Clients can project intense emotions onto the miniature figures,
which can then safely act out these feelings. It can feel much safer for the client
to project difficult and potentially frightening emotions onto miniature people
or animals than it would be to verbalize them. This therapeutic distance creates a greater sense of safety.

4. *Displacement*: Clients can displace negative feelings onto the miniatures
rather than expressing them directly toward family members. Sandtray therapy
provides not only the opportunity for abreaction to occur, but facilitates the
process through the setting, the media, and the process.

Gil (2012) summarizes these dynamics, suggesting that sandtray therapy:

allows for externalized creations of internal 'worlds' of affect, cognitions, perceptions,
picture memories, and compartmentalized aspects of difficult life experiences. This therapy allows for mental and physical assimilation, access to symbol language and metaphor, and the possibility of both chronicling events (creating narrative scenarios), and
utilizing a type of guided imagery that can promote insight and change. (p. 256)

Traumatized clients need the safety of sandtray to explore and express these "internal
worlds."

NEUROBIOLOGICAL EFFECTS OF TRAUMA

Sandtray therapy has significant potential to positively impact the psychology and neurobiology of traumatized clients. As opposed to the limited focus that verbally based interventions have on the executive functioning of the cortical area of the brain, which has limited
ability to process trauma (van der Kolk, 2014)—sandtray work creates a nonverbally
based, experiential, and sensory experience, to process deeper neurobiological issues.

Trauma can eventuate in significant neurobiological activity. There is an increased
production of catecholamines (e.g., epinephrine and norepinephrine) which results in
increased sympathetic nervous system activity (where the fight/flight/freeze response
is located). There are often decreased levels of corticosteroids and serotonin, the most
pronounced effect probably being the decreased ability to moderate the catecholamine-
triggered fight/flight/freeze response. Additionally, there are increased levels of endog-
enous opioids, which may result in pain reduction, emotional blunting, and memory
impairment. It is important to realize that chronic exposure to traumatic stress effects
the adaptation of these chemicals. In other words, it may permanently alter how people
deal with their environment on a daily basis.

A specific example of this neurobiological affect of trauma might be seen in limbic
system activity. The limbic system is the part of the central nervous system that guides
emotion, memory, and behavior necessary for self-preservation. Trauma may cause
limbic system abnormalities in the amygdala and hippocampus. The amygdala, which
readies the body for action, may get 'hijacked' by these neurobiological changes, and
the trauma victim responds before the 'thinking' part of the brain (i.e., cerebral cortex)
can identify threats. The resultant hypervigilance seen in trauma victims can cause
them to go immediately from stimulus to an arousal response, without being able to
make the intervening assessment of the source of their arousal. This causes them to
overreact and intimidate others.

Trauma affects many other parts of the brain as well. The hypothalamic-pituitary-
adrenal (HPA) axis is very vulnerable to stress, as are various noradrenergic systems.

MRI scans of abused and neglected clients show evidence of cortical atrophy or ventricular enlargement. For example, in research of child subjects with PTSD, there is evidence of broad neuronal atrophy and diminished development (De Bellis & Zisk, 2014). This includes smaller intracranial, cerebral, prefrontal cortex, prefrontal cortical white matter, right temporal lobe volumes, and areas of the corpus callosum and its sub-regions. Don't get lost in the big words, however! The bottom line is that research shows that a pattern of atrophy (shrinkage) can be pervasive in the brain. There can be a slowing of brain development, and a reduction of existing brain volume (size).

Because of the excess and adverse neurobiological results of trauma, people with PTSD may experience a deactivation of the prefrontal cortex, which is responsible for executive function. This interferes with their ability to measure and respond to threats. This not only makes navigating post-trauma life difficult, but also interferes with the therapeutic process: High levels of emotional and physiological arousal are occurring, but the ability to process these is hampered. Van der Kolk (2002) notes: "Trauma by definition involves *speechless terror*: patients often are simply unable to put what they feel into words and are left with intense emotions simply without being able to articulate what is going on" (p. 150).

> Trauma by definition involves speechless terror: patients often are simply unable to put what they feel into words and are left with intense emotions without being able to articulate what is going on (van der Kolk, 2002, p. 150).

This has been demonstrated in several neuroimaging studies (Carrion, Wong, & Kletter, 2013; De Bellis & Zisk, 2014; Lanius et al., 2004). For example, when people with PTSD relive their traumatic experience, which is what we ask them to do in therapy, there is decreased activity in Broca's area of the brain, which is related to language. At the same time, there is increased activity in the limbic system, or emotional responses (van der Kolk, 2014). When traumatized people are reliving their trauma, they have great difficulty verbalizing these experiences. This is indeed *speechless terror.*

Perry (2009) argues that for clients to experience change, perhaps even reversal of the compiled neural erosion of damaged attachment and trauma, interventions must target underdeveloped and corrupted regions of the brain. This is particularly important in the regions most impacted by trauma, including self-regulation, executive functioning, relational connection, sensory integration, and memory. To resolve and reform dysfunctional neural networks, interventions must activate these systems (Gaskill & Perry, 2012, 2014; Perry, 2009). Perry (2006) encapsulates this: "Matching the correct therapeutic activities to the specific developmental stage and physiological needs of a maltreated or traumatized child is a key to success" (p. 29). We assert that sandtray therapy can provide this.

Badenoch and Kestly (2015) provide an important summary of the neurological benefits of play and sandtray experiences as they relate to trauma work:

> What most needs to change is the embodied subjective sense within the implicit memory, since that is what continues to come into the present, bringing perceptions, feelings and behaviors with it. . . . It appears that the neural nets holding implicit memory open to new information when two conditions are met: The implicit memory is alive in the body and it is met with what is called a disconfirming experience. That is, the implicit memory is met with an embodied experience of what was missing and needed at the time of the original event . . . In the context of a play therapy relationship that is intent on being alive to the present moment, it is possible for these disconfirming experiences to unfold in the moment-to-moment relational interchange surrounding the arising of these implicit memories. (pp. 528–529)

As noted in Chapter 5, we often use the sandtray creation as a springboard for therapist-client interaction and discussion. This, itself, has neurological benefit. Badenoch (2008) encourages discussion of the tray's meaning with the client, stating that "in terms of brain integration, talking about the tray at this stage can help foster connection between the hemispheres by adding words to the rich experience that has unfolded nonverbally" (p. 224). This *hemispherical* perspective is echoed by Siegel (2003): "To have a coherent story, the drive of the left to tell a logical story must draw on the information from the right. If there is a blockage, as occurs in PTSD, then the narrative may be incoherent" (p. 15).

Badenoch (2008) also suggests that it is helpful to inquire about the feeling of the tray, as opposed to looking for cognitive meaning: "We don't want to catalyze a leap from right- to left-hemisphere processes, but rather open the highway for the right to offer itself to the left" (p. 224). This is supported by Gaskill and Perry (2012), who assert that as "neural activity is transmitted to higher, more complex areas (limbic and cortical), more intricate cognitive associations are made, allowing interpretation of the experience" (p. 33). This should be a reminder to sandtray therapists that interpretation should be left to the client, for both emotional and neurobiological purposes.

At the same time, it is important to be sensitive to the fact that too much inquiry may well defeat the purpose for using sandtray therapy—providing a nonverbally-based intervention, so that a sense of safety can be maintained through a facilitative process. This is in opposition to the potentially intrusive nature of the standard Socratic nature of verbal therapy.

Sandtray therapy is particularly suited to the limbic and neocortical areas of brain development. In Perry's (2006) model of *Sequential Neurodevelopment and Therapeutic Activity* (p. 41), play therapy and storytelling—primary elements of sandtray therapy—are the primary therapeutic and enrichment activities for the limbic and cortex brain areas.

Traumatized clients benefit from an intervention that can be calming and soothing. As noted above, trauma can leave the client's brain in an alarm state, where alarm reactions trump cortical processing (Perry, 2006; van der Kolk, 2006, 2014). The cortical areas of the brain can be overwhelmed by lower regions of the brain, thus an intervention such as sandtray therapy—which does not exclusively rely on verbal processing and executive functioning—helps to sooth clients who may have alarm reactions in the therapy process. Perry and Hambrick (as cited in Gaskill & Perry, 2012) emphasize that "until state regulation or healthy homeostasis is established at the brainstem level, higher brain mediated treatments will be less effective" (p. 40).

In the *Neurosequential Model of Therapeutics* developed by Dr. Bruce Perry (Gaskill & Perry, 2012, 2014; Perry, 2006, 2009), it is suggested that therapy with traumatized and children—as well as traumatized adolescents and adults—begin with a focus on the lower brain regions [the brainstem and diencephalon (mid-brain)] and work upwards. This would include moving through the higher brains areas identified by Perry as the limbic and cortical areas. Perry (2009) posits:

> Once there is improvement in self-regulation, the therapeutic work can move to more relational-related problems (limbic) using more traditional play or arts therapies; ultimately, once fundamental dyadic relational skills have improved, the therapeutic techniques can be more verbal and insight oriented (cortical) using any variety of cognitive-behavioral or psychodynamic approach. (p. 252)

We would assert that sandtray therapy follows this very progression. The initial therapeutic work, from the very first touching of the sand, is fundamentally brainstem- and diencephalon-related. Badenoch (2008) asserts that arranging the sand is an experience that "encourages vertical integration, linking body, limbic region, and cortex in the right hemisphere" (p. 223). This sand play focuses on the tactile, motor, and attunement needed for the brainstem—as well as the rhythmic, simple narrative and physical warmth needed for the diencephalon (see Perry, 2006). Sandtray work can then bring a client to the relational and narrative elements of play therapy needed for the limbic area, moving to the narrative and conversational [as well as insight] needed for the cortex (Perry). Badenoch (2008) also speaks to this, stating: "Grounded in the body, sandplay unfolds through the limbic regions and cortex and spans both hemispheres as the symbolic world unfolds into words" (p. 220). Sandtray therapy begins with the basic materials of sand and miniature figures, thus having an initial focus on the lower stress-response networks, before moving on to cognitive and relational interactions through the processing of sandtray creations.

IMPACT ON THERAPEUTIC PROCESS

For therapists who rely solely on verbal interventions, many of the fundamental neurobiological results of trauma are being ignored. Van der Kolk (as cited in Wylie, 2004) speaks to this:

> Fundamentally, words can't integrate the disorganized sensations and action patterns that form the core imprint of the trauma. . . . To do effective therapy, we need to do things that change the way people regulate these core functions, which probably can't be done by words and language alone. (p. 38)

We would posit that sandtray therapy meets this goal.

In regard to the difficulty (or impossibility) of putting the trauma narrative into words, Malchiodi (2015) suggests an important insight and rationale for an expressive intervention such as sandtray therapy:

> Perhaps this inability to verbalize one's response to trauma relates to the human survival response; when an experience is extremely painful to recall, the brain protects the individual by literally making it impossible to talk about it. Because trauma is stored as somatic sensations and images, it may not be readily available for communication through language, but may be available through sensory means such as creative arts, play, and other experiential activities and approaches. (p. 11)

If therapists focus primarily on the emotionally charged content of the trauma, a client's fundamental physiological state can shift. Perry (2006) suggests that this shift may lead to the client and the therapy becoming "brainstem-driven" (p. 34). The resultant anxiety, in addition to the possible diminished functioning of Broca's area, leads clients to act in a primitive manner. This renders the verbal language of therapy less accessible, or perhaps useless: "No matter how much you talk to someone, the words will not easily get translated into changes in the midbrain or the brain stem" (Perry & Pate, 1994, p. 141).

The implications for therapy are obvious. That is, traditional verbal therapy may well be ineffective, and perhaps detrimental. This is not to eschew cognitively based interventions. Rather, therapists must be cross-trained in expressive (nonverbally based) therapies in order to access trauma in clients, which is frequently based in the midbrain as opposed to the executive neurological areas. Sandtray therapy is a particularly effective expressive medium, which is used with trauma victims of all ages.

The operation of brain hemispheres and the hemispheric results of trauma also point to the need for an intervention such as sandtray therapy. Gil (2006) notes that evidence "suggests that trauma memories are imbedded in the right hemisphere of the brain . . . thus that interventions facilitating access to and activity in the right side of the brain may be indicated" (p. 68). Sandtray therapy is one of these. Badenoch (2008) states that sandtray has a "notable ability to awaken and then regulate right-brain limbic processes [which] can make it a powerful way to address painful, fearful, dissociated experiences" (p. 220).

An awareness of the operation of the brain hemispheres is therapeutically important. The right hemisphere is more focused on the nonverbal, artistic, and metaphorical. The left hemisphere, by contrast, is focused more upon linear processing. The integration of the hemispheres is important for normal functioning, and appears to be negatively impacted by trauma. Specifically, trauma precipitates abnormalities in the corpus callosum, the fiber tract connecting the two hemispheres (Teicher, Tomoda, & Andersen, 2006). This may explain the challenges in lateralization (accessing both hemispheres) that abused clients sometimes experience, and can certainly affect the narrative of the trauma.

Sandtray therapy avoids the typical treatment dynamic, which expects clients to express the narrative of their traumatic experience in words. Verbal therapy tends to be linear in nature. Siegel (2003) speaks to the inherent challenges in this:

> The linear telling of a story is driven by the left hemisphere. In order to be autobiographical, the left side must connect with the subjective emotional experience that is stored in the right hemisphere. The proposal is this: to have a coherent story, the drive of the left to tell a logical story must draw on the information from the right. If there is a blockage, as occurs in PTSD, then the narrative may be incoherent. . . . When one achieves neural integration across the hemispheres, one achieves coherent narratives. (p. 15)

Our proposal is this: Providing a nonverbally based expressive medium such as sandtray reaches the metaphorically focused right hemisphere. Therefore, accessing and expressing the traumatic narrative is enhanced. While we endorse the benefit of expressing the trauma narrative, it does not have to be (and indeed sometimes cannot be) verbal in nature. As noted above, it may be more advantageous to focus on feeling, rather than looking at cognitive meaning, opening the "highway for the right to offer itself to the left" (Badenoch, 2008, p. 224).

Too many therapists, well trained in their area of expertise, do not recognize the need to consider these neurobiological effects. Perry (2006) notes

> Simply stated, traumatic and neglectful experiences . . . cause abnormal organization and function of important neural systems in the brain, compromising the functional capacities mediated by these systems. . . . Matching the correct therapeutic activities to the specific developmental stage and physiological needs of a maltreated or traumatized child is the key to success. (p. 29)

This is true for adults as well.

According to Rothbaum and Foa (1996), there are two basic conditions needed in therapy for the reduction of fear, and thus the treatment of PTSD: (1) the person must attend to trauma-related material in a way that will activate traumatic memories, and (2) the context (the therapeutic process) needs to directly contradict the major elements of the trauma, primarily feeling safe. Safety may, in fact, be the crucial factor in treating traumatized clients. Trauma victims don't just feel psychologically unsafe, but also neurobiologically unsafe. The sandtray therapy process meets these two conditions.

Additionally, the relational safety in the sandtray therapy process provides an important element of trauma treatment. Recognizing that therapeutic growth cannot occur outside of the scope of intrapersonal and interpersonal safety, the expressive and projective nature of sandtray promotes this needed element. Van der Kolk (2006) discusses a key aspect of this dynamic:

> While human contact and attunement are cardinal elements of physiological self-regulation, interpersonal trauma often results in a fear of intimacy. The promise of closeness and attunement for many traumatized individuals automatically evokes implicit

memories of hurt, betrayal, and abandonment. As a result, feeling seen and understood, which ordinarily helps people to feel a greater sense of calm and in control, may precipitate a reliving of the trauma . . . this means that, as trust is established it is critical to help create a physical sense of control by working on the establishment of physical boundaries. (p. 289)

As noted earlier, the sandtray is the *container* of the client's psyche, and the sandtray therapist has the role of being a facilitator and witness to the clients' telling and processing of their presenting issue. This facilitates the development of the needed control, for which van der Kolk is arguing. Additionally, the client's sense of feeling seen and understood unfolds in a way that is less threatening through sandtray therapy, as sandtray therapists honor the creation and processing of the sandtray without the transference and countertransference that may occur with other therapeutic modalities.

GOAL OF SANDTRAY WITH TRAUMATIZED CLIENTS

Our first goal in treating traumatized clients through sandtray therapy is to provide clients with a safe, reparative, and relational experience. This takes priority over a focus on insight and/or cognitive restructuring. The meaning of the trauma to the client may be important, but not as important as processing it so that it can become tolerable and manageable. After this occurs, meaning can then be sought. Our roles, therefore, are primarily to be fellow sojourners on the journey and witnesses to the clients' stories.

If clients are unable to talk about their trauma, they will have the symptomatic response, but essentially no story. The trauma has expression, but only through recreation of the trauma, resulting in internal, external, and/or relational impairment. The task of therapeutic interventions should be to return control to clients and help them develop a sense of mastery. Sandtray therapy reaches through the psychological and neurobiological obstacles to assist in this process, and helps clients develop their narrative and begin a new story.

An example of a typical trauma-focused intervention would be a cognitive restructuring treatment, focused on the use of *Socratic dialogue*. One illustration is provided by Monson and Shnaider (2014), who suggest cognitive techniques such as

Clarifying Questions: Who was there at the time? What did they do? What happened just before? Afterward? What were you thinking and feeling at the time?

Challenging Assumptions: What other things could have happened had you done something differently? Have you ever met a good person who had bad things happen to them? What information did you have at the time of the event, not now that the event is over?

Evaluating Objective Evidence: What is the probability of _____ (safety concern) in your current circumstances? Do you know of at least one exception to your current conclusion?

Challenging Underlying or Core Beliefs: What would it mean if you didn't blame yourself for what happened? (p. 55)

These may be effective for some clients, with the assumption that they have the psychological and neurobiological resources to interact around these questions. If they do not, perhaps due to some of the dynamics discussed above, we would suggest incorporating sandtray therapy. Sandtray therapy could be used as an adaption of these questions—perhaps using miniature figures to pose or answer these questions—or using sandtray as a means to provide safety in preparation for using such a directive and cognitive approach.

The trauma narrative does need to be processed. It is possible, and we would argue, beneficial—that this trauma narrative develop with the context of an expressive and projective intervention such as sandtray therapy. This perspective is shared by several sandtray therapists (Duffy, 2015; Kestly, 2014; Lacroix et al., 2007; McCarthy, 2006; Miller & Boe, 1990; Raftopoulos, 2015). This provides the safe, reparative, and relational experience we hope to provide with traumatized clients.

11

Assessment Across the Ages
Developmental Norms and Diagnostic Signs and Indicators

Understanding the techniques and methods we use is fundamental to both effective assessment and intervention. Setting the example, Margaret Lowenfeld studied her new form of clinical work with children (Lowenfeld, 1939, 1979a). As the clinical experience with children further developed, the use of the World and the number of children using it grew, Lowenfeld discovered *basic symptoms* common in their work. Lowenfeld identified these as: (a) fencing, in large parts of the children's worlds; (b) wild animals, placed where they do not belong; (c) frequent recurrence of the same miniature figures; and (d) placement of other miniature figures where they do not belong. Lowenfeld did not pursue statistical analysis of her findings, compare her child clients with non-clinical children, nor researched to develop normative data (Bühler, 1951a, 1951b). Rather, Lowenfeld's focus was on the development of a form of communication for children.

Charlotte Bühler (1951a, 1951b), a child development theorist and researcher and contemporary of Lowenfeld, became inquisitive in the usefulness of Lowenfeld's World Technique materials for the establishing of developmental norms and the ability to assess clinical symptoms. Bühler's subsequent *World Test* included a standardized set of 160 miniature figures (she called *elements*) for her quantitative research, or a box of 300 for qualitative research and therapeutic use. These miniature figures were organized by category in separate compartments in a box to be used by the research subjects in a six-foot square space on the floor or a table. Bühler stated this is "a way the World material can be used in play therapy . . . The World material is diagnostically informative and serves as the beginning of a therapeutic experience for the child" (Bühler, 1951b, p. 75).

Hanna Bratt, a Swedish educator, became aware of the World Technique and was intrigued in its use as a therapeutic and communicative technique with children. Bratt studied with Lowenfeld in 1933 and went on to develop *The Sandtray*, the Swedish version of The World Technique (Nelson, 2011). Bratt expanded her clinical work and in 1934 established the Erica Foundation, where The Sandtray was used therapeutically with children 4 to 12 years of age (p. 826). In the mid-1940s the Erica Foundation began to use The Sandtray for diagnostic purposes under the leadership of Gösta Harding. While continuing to develop The Sandtray for diagnostic purposes, Harding integrated the various age-level, developmental work of Bühler and added the psychoanalytic libido-development perspective (Nelson, 2011). However, in therapeutic work, he stated, "We do not theorize so much here—we must live intensively with the child from day to day, and as a gardener looks at his flowers, see how it is growing and developing" (Nelson, 2011, p. 831). Finally, Allis Danielson, inspired by Harding, further expanding The Sandtray as a diagnostic instrument and in his manual of the same name, *The Erica Method*, it became the name under which it is now known (Nelson, 2011, pp. 831–832).

DEVELOPMENTAL NORMS

What do normal, non-clinical individuals, children through older adults, build in the sand tray? How do we as clinicians identify the 'clinical' in the tray from the 'non-clinical' and age-appropriate creations in the tray? These seem to be important questions to explore.

Just as a clinicians who uses art in therapy is familiar with what regressed art work looks like, or aware of indicators in the art work for clinical issues, they have an understanding of age appropriate drawing in which to base these decisions. Child development specialists use play to assess children, also based on the typical play for a given age. Sandtray therapists can do the same (roughly speaking!). Over time, several researchers and sandtray therapists have studied the typical, non-clinical creations in the trays of various age groups. As indicated above, Charlotte Bühler, Hanna Bratt, Gösta Harding, Allis Danielson, and likely others, explored developmental norms grounded in Margaret Lowenfeld's work. A few additional researchers, more current to this era, have done the same, either looking at developmental norms, or researching clinical groups alongside non-clinical control groups. These studies continue to inform our understanding of normal play in the sand tray. These include Bower (1970), Burke (1996), Cockle (1993), Grubbs (1995), Harper (1991), Jones (1986), Mattson and Veldorale-Brogan (2010), Mitchell and Friedman (1994), Petruk (1996), Werner (1956), and Zunni (1997), among others. Cherrie Glasse (1995), a school teacher and then a clinical psychologist, connected characteristics of sand tray creations with Piaget's (1951) cognitive stages. Given most clinicians familiarity with Piaget's work, we will also use Piaget's stages to organize the normative findings. Appendix C is a Sand Tray Assessment Worksheet to use in reviewing sand tray creations using the following researched-based information.

Below is a compilation of the characteristics of sand tray constructions found in the research studies mentioned above. They are organized by Piaget's cognitive developmental stages, for the ease of the clinician seeking to identify age-typical components. A caveat: We caution the reader about the information below. It is accumulated from several studies, none of which have a large subject pool, except perhaps Bühler's. Many findings support each other. Also, when seeking to identify 'what is normal' we need to remember that all developmental levels include a range of behavior or indicators as well as outliers.

PREOPERATIONAL—INTUITIVE COGNITIVE STAGE, AGES 2–7

This stage is marked by thinking which is based on intuition and is still not completely logical. Children are able to represent things with words, symbols, images and as they age, use letters and numbers. Children use pretend play, are egocentric, and language development soars during these years.

Use of sand

- Pushes, pours
- Buries/unburies, ages 2–3
- one to two small bodies of water, small pond, partial river

- Vehicle tracks
- Roads with unclear destination or connection
- Patted mounds

Boundaries

Created by use of sand and figure groupings

☐ Sense of boundaries, primitive quality and lack of clarity, incomplete paths, ponds, lakes, mounds

☐ May appear without intentionality, ages 2–3

☐ Very simple: line/rows of soldiers, or other items, increasing with ages 5–8

Created by typical boundary figures

☐ Limited or primitive

Disrupted by anomalies

☐ Create a scattered effect or disrupt the theme

Use of miniature figures

☐ 0–1 yrs., ≤ 25% of tray used and figures placed outside tray.

☐ 2–3 yrs., most of tray used, but not uncommon to use only part; figures within tray; places figures on front horizontal edge and left corner; play with figures on floor; may throw or poke into sand; pour sand over people; doesn't exhibit control—chaotic worlds; figures prone, jungle animals; eating themes.

☐ 3–4 yrs., builds scenes with increased coherent detail.

☐ 4–5 yrs., figures placed along one horizontal edge and one corner, also in intervals across the tray area.

☐ 4–6 yrs., engaged in dramatic activity (making zooming noises with airplanes).

☐ 4–8 yrs., 91–100% of tray used; all figures within the tray; all used people and cars; increasing use of rows; dramatic play with animal figures and vehicles.

☐ 5 yrs. and above, arranged figures in groups, use all four sides of tray; mean/average number of figures 50–70.

Orientation and Relationship of Human Figures

☐ Side-by-side; in front of, behind one another.

☐ Dyads; human or animal families.

☐ If two or more human figures, in a dramatic grouping; dramatic play with human figures.

☐ Beginning of relationships—two or more figures purposefully oriented, interpersonally and functionally related.

☐ By age 5 yrs., small constructions (example: house, fenced with people and trees).

Worldview: Observation of How Complicated and Coherent the Theme

☐ Suggestion of differentiated perspectives, but are either a single underdeveloped theme alone, or several unrelated themes.

☐ Ages 4–5 exhibit preoccupation with having enough food for people and animals.

CONCRETE OPERATIONS COGNITIVE STAGE, AGES 7–11

Children in this stage are able to think logically about concrete events and ask about concrete analogies. Thinking is now marked with conservation, reversibility, serial ordering, and a mature understanding of cause-and-effect. Keeping rules is important.

Use of sand

- Rivers runs side-to-side.
- Medium lakes, more than two bodies of water.
- Clear roads; hills and mountains, islands, valleys, roads, waves, furrows volcanoes, sand walls and rarely seen in younger children.
- Figures, faces drawn.

Boundaries

Created by use of sand and figure grouping

- ☐ Goal lines, furrows, diagrams, lakes with islands.
- ☐ Boundaries that are simple and moderately clear.
- ☐ Rivers not completely delineated.
- ☐ Well-coordinated groups that are complex.

Created by typical boundary figures

- ☐ Appropriate use, moderately clear and without primitive quality.
- ☐ Paths, roads, signs; fences are defined by rocks and/or hedges, bridges, etc.
- ☐ Obvious connections within the sand world.

Disrupted by anomalies

- ☐ Not seriously impinging on clear boundaries but are intrusive.

Use of miniature figures

- ☐ 91–100% of tray is used; all figures are within confines of the tray; no barren or empty trays.
- ☐ 47% of those in this age group used water.
- ☐ Number of miniatures used increases concurrently with increasing age; younger children used average of 64 figures.
- ☐ Includes number of trees.

Orientation and relationship of human figures

- ☐ On top of one another, inside, seated, supine/lying flat.
- ☐ Parts of community (bands, neighborhood).
- ☐ Played out cowboy and Indians themes, opposing forces being apparent.
- ☐ Dramatic action between figures obvious by placement; action relationship between figures.
- ☐ Boys: themes of adversity and struggle, resolved threats and conflicts.
- ☐ Girls: religious and spiritual themes; dyadic interactions; family relationships.
- ☐ Dramatic play decreases with age.

Worldview: observation of how complicated and coherent the theme

- ☐ Construction created with a basic plan that is then filled in with details; typically the initial layout includes houses, fences, or bridges.

□ Sets of object-groups in simple concrete, single-themed; uniting simple parts.

□ If parts are complex, there is a scattered, step-by-step quality.

□ Constructs of peaceful farm scenes.

Formal Operational Cognitive Stage, Ages 11 and Up

This stage is marked with the ability to think about hypothetical scenarios and the ability to process abstract thoughts, abstract logic, deductive reasoning, comparison, and classification. Has potential for mature moral reasoning; awareness of complex emotions.

Use of sand

■ Diagonal, winding rivers, with delineated source in lake or spring, and runs into lake or ocean.

■ Roads with clear destinations and connections.

■ Cliffs, pits, dens, tunnels, land bridges.

■ Pyramids, castles, mines, graves.

Boundaries

Created by use of sand and figure groupings

□ Oceans and/or clearly delineated rivers, roads, various combinations of bodies of water, hills, pits, mountains.

□ Unusual formations that create clear boundaries that also united the world.

□ Complex grouping in a unified relationship forming the boundaries that both unify and separate, allowing a complexity of parts to be a part of the whole.

Created by typical boundary figures

□ Complex and clear relationship creating a sense of boundaries that both separates and unifies complex parts.

□ Created by well-coordinated groupings which may relate to complex world.

Disrupted by anomalies

□ Nothing abnormal in the sand world.

Use of miniature figures

□ 91–100% of tray used; all are within confines of the tray.

□ No dramatic play; but could be placed in creative way to show dramatic movement.

□ Frequently includes trees.

□ Typically constructed scene of town or village which includes school, church (or both), or landscape along with a human settlement.

Orientation and relationship of human figures

□ Orientation: Under other figures (trees, bridges); entering into or emerging from buildings; complex configurations (football games, town destroyed in battle).

□ Relationship: Whole animal/human communities, clearly defined and integrated.

□ Figures displaying the human community are clearly established or integrated, lone figure may be used.

Worldview: observation of how complicated and coherent the theme

- ☐ Coherent, symbolic or abstract or differentiated realistic world.
- ☐ Concepts such as "native land," social justice, religion.
- ☐ Single, coherent overview such as humor or spirituality uniting parts that might otherwise seem unrelated.
- ☐ Single, clearly recognizable thematic overview uniting complex parts which are interdependent and integrated.
- ☐ Symbolic and realistic worlds created and characterized by a single theme encompassing complex parts that may not be completely integrated.

OTHER STUDIES WITH ADULTS: 21–65 YEARS

- ■ 10 minutes, average, time to build
- ■ Feels sand and sculpts it, no use of tools
- ■ Number of figures used (inconsistent findings):
   - ☐ Average 15 figures (Mattson & Veldorale-Brogan, 2010)
   - ☐ Over 100 (Bowyer, 1970)
- ■ Distributed to all areas of the tray
- ■ Frequent use of houses and trees
- ■ Scenes from their past; may appear to regress

The above compilation of normative information from various research studies certainly is not fully comprehensive. We do hope that this gathering of the information which has been located and reviewed, together in one place, will be useful to you in your sand tray work.

Diagnostic Indicators and Signs in the Sand Tray

Empirical research in the area of assessment of diagnostic indicators or signs in sand tray work is minimal. Developmental studies began with Charlotte Bühler's pioneering work in 1934 (as cited in Bradway et al., 1981, p. 9) later shifted to diagnostic assessment. Bühler named her diagnostic technique the *World Test* and later to the *Toy World Test* (1951a). She did find significant differences between clinical and nonclinical populations, but could not differentiate diagnoses within the clinical group (later research supports this inability to identify diagnosis by a sandtray construction). Bühler compared worlds created by 174 children from Vienna, London, Oslo, Holland, and the United States. She scored the trays by number of items used, types of items used or omitted, and the arrangement in the tray. The arrangement was identified by disorder or order, schematic or realistic, and scattered or closed. Bühler subsequently identified seven characteristics identifying those in need of clinical services:

1. fewer than 50 items;
2. five or fewer categories of items;
3. avoiding use of men or women;
4. use of aggressive items (soldiers, wild animal attacks, etc.);
5. closed world, where most of the construction is fenced in;
6. worlds with rows of items, over exaggerated uniformity; and
7. disorganized worlds, chaotic placement.

Bühler indicated that two or more characteristics (identifiers) have to be found for the tray to be identified as an indication of emotional disturbance. She noted that one characteristic can be found in trays of nonclinical individuals.

Other researchers who followed found the same ability to differentiate clinical from nonclinical groups (Fujii, 1979; Harper, 1991; Lumry, 1951; Mitchell & Friedman, 1994; Petruk, 1996). Lumry (1951) assessed sand tray worlds of children classified as normal, stutterers, withdrawn, or retarded. Each group had 25 children, 6.5 to 9.5 years of age. None of the 25 children in the normal group showed more than one of Bühler's diagnostic characteristics, supporting the earlier findings. Only 3 of the 75 other children displayed none of the diagnostic characteristics in their sand tray worlds. Lumry's study was unable to differentiate among the three clinical groups supporting Bühler's findings.

Fujii (1979) studied 20 normal, delinquent, or emotionally disturbed 10 to 14 year old boys. The boys made two trays, 2 to 3 weeks apart. Eight to 10 judges were able to identify the trays built by either the delinquent or emotionally disturbed boys (inter-rater reliability, $p = .001$).

Petruk's (1996) descriptive study compared nonclinical children with those who were living in a children's shelter, having been removed from their home by Children Protective Services. She also sought to discover if children could be correctly identified as being in need of mental health services by their first sandtray construction. Petruk had 20 nonclinical children and eight clinical children, ages 9 to 11, selected to match Piaget's Concrete Operational Stage. The children were invited to "use these miniatures to build or create a world in the sand tray, choose as many or few as you like, . . . I will be sitting over here" (p. 75). The children had 30 minutes to build and then time to tell the story of the sand tray creation. Clinical and nonclinical could be correctly identified by the photographs scored by blind reviewers.

Cockle (1993) compared trays of five coping and five difficulty-coping children ranging in age from 6 years, 11 months, to 8 years, 7 months (second and third graders). Coping children were defined as those who got along well with teachers and peers and displayed average developmental mastery of learning skills. Difficulty-coping children were identified as those who failed to get along with teachers and peers and had failed to master work skills necessary for their grade level. The children each made four trays each over 2 months. The child had access to a dry tray and a damp tray along with miniatures. The children were invited to make a "picture or scene in the sand using any of the miniature articles they wished" during a 30-minute session (Cockle, 1993, p. 3). Once the tray was completed, the child was asked to describe the creation. Differences in the use of the dry or damp sandtray varied little. However, the coping children (CC) never used both trays in the same session. The difficulty-coping children (DCC) used both trays in the same session 40% of the time. Thematically there were some striking differences. The CC showed safety, empowerment, and dependency themes (15%, 15%, and 25%, respectively) compared to no display of these themes by the DCC. DCC showed themes of struggle (40% to 5% by CC), death/destruction (25% to 5%), and danger/threat (20% to 5%; pp. 12–13).

These are examples of research that looked at the differences between clinical and nonclinical individuals. There has not been sufficient research, nor sufficient sample sizes, to validate a diagnostic instrument. The largest and most useful, perhaps, is Bühler's (1951a, 1951b) and her findings are supported by later research studies. As stated earlier, Bühler indicated two or more of her indicators identify the need for clinical intervention. The following list and organization of the clinical indicators is adapted from Bühler's (1951b) scoring form for the World Test and may be useful clinically, if not diagnostically. Also, as a reminder, nonclinical individuals frequently had one indicator.

Bühler's Clinical Indicators

Aggressive Worlds

1. Soldiers fighting
2. Animals biting, wild animals fighting
3. Accidents (fires, crashing, killing, burying, robbery)

Empty Worlds

4. Fewer than 50 miniature figures (individuals 8 years and over)
5. Fewer than 5 categories (individuals 7 years and over)
6. Men and women omitted

Distorted Worlds

7. Closed/fenced (individuals 5 years and over)
     Many small enclosed areas; total or nearly total enclosed areas
8. Disorganized (individuals 5 years and over)
     Odd placements; disconnected; chaotic
9. Rigid (individuals 6 yrs. and over)
     Schematic; rows

These are also located on the Sand Tray Assessment Worksheet (Appendix C). We have found that recognition of these clinical indicators, and the possible meaning of them for the client, are particularly useful for those new to the use of the sand tray (as discussed in Chapter 5). Awareness of these possible indicators can assist the novice sandtray therapist formulate therapeutically focused questions during the processing portion of the sand tray session. Of course, all session formats and questions are tailored to the specific theoretical approach of the sandtray therapist.

CONCLUSION

Many clinicians who add a sandtray experience with clients are often amazed at the depth of work and meaningfulness of the sessions to the clients and their understanding of their clients. Therefore, many clinicians unfortunately jump into working with the sand tray without, in our view, sufficient understanding of it. As mentioned in other sections of this book, ethical concerns about education, training, and supervision are paramount. Also, is the understanding of developmental norms, as based in a long history of research, even if not numerous. Understanding age-appropriate, typical work with miniature figures in the sand tray, adds to our knowledge base which in turn, helps our work be more powerful and ethical. Knowing the possible clinical indicators likewise informs our practice.

12

Research

Research of the use of sandtray therapy in a variety of clinical settings is increasing. This logically follows the continued considerable growth in its use by mental health professionals. Research is critical to inform our practice. It provides an understanding of the process, as well as a level of efficacy as a treatment intervention. Research, along with case studies and theoretical pieces, build the body of literature upon which a modality is based. The sandtray therapy literature began with Lowenfeld's World Technique (1950) and Kalff's Sandplay (1980). It continues through many venues and writers. Well-designed and executed research studies are critical. In the current mental health care climate, outcome-studies upon which to base treatment that is proven to be effective, is critical. Evidence-based treatment is not currently available in the sandtray therapy arena. What we do have is empirical research that informs our best practices. A selection of those research studies will be described here. These studies can inform how you use the sandtray therapy process with your clients, assist you in communicating its effectiveness to clients, parents of child-clients, and other professionals. We hope it may also challenge researchers to replicate studies, which becomes the basis to obtain evidence-based status. For this to be possible, Ray (2006) challenges researchers to also develop manualized treatment with clear protocols. Published research results must contain a clear reporting of the sample population demographics, including more specific identification of mental health issues. Overgeneralization and use of categories such as 'acting out' is no longer sufficient.

Homeyer and Morrison (2008) challenged practitioners and researchers to remember that there are still philosophical questions regarding what makes treatment effective. Wampold (Neill, 2006) suggests the importance of common treatment factors, such as the impact of the therapeutic relationship between client and therapist, the therapist's competence and belief in the intervention, and the client's own expectations of hope of change. So, is it theory and manualized treatment protocols, or the common factors, or both? We agree with many others that both perspectives need more substantial, thoughtful, innovative, and well-designed, replicable, research.

The research studies are organized by general categories for the reader's convenience. Each study will include a brief description of the purpose of the study and research design, the demographics and selection process of the subjects, the intervention or procedure, and highlights of the results. Studies have numerous and detailed results and an attempt to report all the findings is beyond the scope of this chapter. We have reported effect sizes when available. The Cohen's d effect size is the current preferred method of reporting change. So, when available, the effect size is given. As a reminder, according to Cohen (1988, $d = .2$ represents a small effect size; $d = .5$ is a medium effect size, and $d = .8$ is a large effect size. We highly encourage the reader to read the original research of those studies that intrigue you.

GROUP SANDTRAY THERAPY

Group sandtray therapy is widely used and research on its use is growing. Hughes (2004) and McCown (2008) completed exploratory and descriptive studies, respectfully, to give insight into the process of group sandtray therapy. Both researchers included thoughts regarding the role of the right brain in adjusting the internal working model of self as experienced within the group setting. Brain research (Badenoch, 2008; Schore, 2009; Siegel, 1999) supports these hypotheses. Two strong experiential design research projects (Flahive, 2005; Shen, 2006) show positive results regarding the efficacy of group sandtray therapy.

Hughes (2004) studied a single session of group sand tray. As she indicated, because there was no existing research on the group sand tray process at the time of her research, her study was to generate, rather than test, a hypothesis. The exploratory research question was, "How can psychotherapists and others understand the projective dynamics of a group engaged in a sand tray session?" She used triangulation in her qualitative research analysis of the verbalizations of participants during the group experience, interviews with the participants following the experience, and her own personal reflections. Triangulation was used to ensure and practice empathic neutrality during qualitative research data analysis.

The participants were a convenient sample of three men and eleven women, between the ages of 30 and 65. All participants were either doctorate-level professors or doctoral candidates attending an academic conference on science and creativity during which they participated in this single group sand tray session. The participants used an approximately 2.5-foot-square sandtray on a round table, with miniatures located on another. The recorded session lasted about two hours which was "roughly divided into periods of miniature selection tray building, individual explanations, exchanges of ideas, tray adjustments with vocalizations, discussion, adjustments in silence, discussion, more adjustments with vocalizations, and wrap-up" (Hughes, 2004, p. 81). The report of the research had no mention of any specific prompt or instructions given to the participants regarding what they were to create or build in the sand tray.

The findings suggest that engaging the right-brain hemisphere consciously and unconsciously (proprioceptively) results in "emerging shared meanings" with the developing culture dynamics. Hughes (2004) stated the "group sand tray itself is a microcosmic description of the prevailing psyche of the culture" (p. 76). Hughes stated that the findings suggest the group experience can increase sharing insight by the participants and improve relational dynamics in the general culture of those involved.

Another one-session group sand tray research project supports the cultural impact of the participants revealed in the created sandtray. Katz (2010) used a large group sand tray in Israel with an existing, ongoing Israeli-Jew and Palestinian-Israeli-Arab encounter group who reflected the "recapitulating the basic Israeli conflict over contested land the sand tray represented" (p. 116). The tray was to "reflect a 'contained' piece of land in which to create their 'shared' world using miniatures" (p. 113). The purpose of the experience was to explore if this very concrete task could influence aspects of their cultural and national conflicts. Trays were built by dyads to create a shared world. The session began by the group sorting the items into categories. This provided the opportunity for group members to handle and become familiar with the items. The prompt was simply to "build your world." Once the building began, further instructions included that they could use as many miniatures as they desired, add or remove items, and had 20 minutes to complete the task. Final analysis of the trays revealed three patterns: Struggle to asset one's self (covert conflict), dominance and submission, and co-existence (p. 117). Katz indicated that the experience "provided each person to see a reflection of their issues of living in a shared space in a safe forum that can foster greater sympathy and compassion for their own conflicts and those of the other" (p. 126).

Multi-family group sand tray experiences to improve the coping skills of parents concerning their adolescents' substance abuse/dependency was studied by James and Martin (2002). These court-ordered groups are open-format with members typically participating 3 to 6 months. Each group consists of seven to ten parents and their adolescent children, aged 13 to 18. A parent completes a tray outside of the group's presence, usually in a counselor's office. The directions are to select figures that show how the parent feels about his/her family, to include figures for self and family members, then using them create a scene in the tray. Once that is complete it is brought into the group room and processed together. James and Martin find that sharing symbolism and themes helps the parents identify patterns of their adolescents' substance-related problems, increase awareness of family relationships while also decreasing denial, reactive anger and stopping enabling behaviors (p. 396).

Roubenzadeh, Abedin, and Heidari (2012) recognize that there are pronounced cultural differences in the resolution of grief and not many models to support this process in Iran. They studied the use of a short-term group sandtray therapy model with 20 grieving youth, 16–22 years old who experienced a death in their family within the past 2 years. This research was a pre-post-test design with a control group. The Grief Experience Inventory (by Bart and Scott; no reference given) provided the data. The findings showed significant reduction in somatic reaction, feelings of guilt and rejection (p. 2131). No between-group analysis was reported in the article.

Children with Autism Spectrum Disorder (ASD) ages 7–12-year-old (23 boys and 2 girls) participated in group sandtray therapy within their special needs classrooms in Canada (Lu, Peterson, Lacroix, & Rousseau, 2010). The children are placed into the classrooms based on age and developmental level; the sandplay took place in their respective classrooms, led by two art therapists. This action research collected data from observation grids, photographs of the sand trays, and teacher observation (p. 59). The students participated in group sandplay in a 60-minute class period once a week for 10 weeks. To establish structured, predictable routine, beneficial for children with ASD each session had an opening group ritual, the sandplay (created in individual trays), storytelling (done, if possible, as a group), and a group closing ritual. Each was session was modified, consistent with action research, to the needs of the particular children. Content analysis provided the following findings. None of the children exhibited negative or regressive behavior during the course of the 10 weeks. There were positive changes in the students' complexification of symbolic use and stories. Students had improved in their general participation and attention. Highly avoidant children progressed from functional play to incorporating symbolic representational play. Some children's rigid play began to show more flexibility, borrowing ideas from their peers sand trays. Other children displayed increased other-awareness, for example, through imitating the placement of miniature figures in their trays, attentive listening to other's stories, and building upon each other's ideas (p. 59). Lu et al. believe that unstructured sandplay provided a "creative space to support the developmental skills of communication, socialization, and symbolic elaboration" (p. 64).

GROUP SANDTRAY THERAPY IN A SCHOOL SETTING

McCown (2008) completed a study of second and third graders in an inclusive sand tray friendship group. Her descriptive study was focused on inclusivity: students with ranges of intellectual and academic functioning, introverted and extroverted, receiving special education services, and both genders. McCown acknowledged the increasing task of schools to serve the growing diversity of students. The purpose of this study was to explore the Sandtray Friendship Group as developed by Kestly (2001, 2010). Kestly also served as a consultant for this research.

Six students, three boys and three girls, participated in this study. They were referred by school staff members. Students were screened out if there were concerns regarding suicide, serious depression, an existing mental health diagnosis, or any previous sand tray group participation. This was a convenient, criterion-based sample, purposefully constructed to be as inclusive of diversity as possible. The group of six students had ten sandtray sessions, two each per week. The students worked in their own individual rectangular tray, in close proximity to each other. Each session had four phases as outlined by Kestly (2001) with some modification to meet the school schedule needs: (1) selection of miniatures, (2) building the trays, (3) students sharing the story of the tray, and (4) closing with a greeting activity. In the final group session students made albums of their sand tray photographs.

Data were collected using observation protocols, guided interview protocols, written feedback from teachers, session protocols, and photographs of all the completed sand trays. Qualitative analysis included coding, themes, and triangulation of the data. Results indicated that the students found the sand tray friendship group was a fun experience. It was a personally unique experience for each student and resulted in improved socialization. Teachers reported improved language and social skills. Teachers specifically noted that participants made new friends and were more outgoing.

Homeyer, Poe and DeFrance (2004) completed a trial study with a boys group and a girls group of fifth graders. A medium effect size was discovered. The groups included students receiving special education as well as others needing counseling services. The structure of the group sandtray therapy sessions followed Kestly's (2001, 2010) the format of individual building of trays, then an invitation for group members to tell the story of the tray.

Preadolescents with behavior difficulties were studied by Flahive (2005) and Flahive & Ray (2007). This was a pretest-posttest control group design. Participants, 9- to 12-years-old and in the fourth or fifth grade, were teacher referred for disruptive behaviors in class, problems getting along with others, symptoms of anxiety or sadness, and withdrawal (p. 367). Fifty-six students were randomly assigned to either the experimental or control group, and were stratified by gender and ethnicity. Members of the experimental group, further divided to treatment groups of three, received sandtray therapy for 10 weeks, while participants in the wait-list control group received no treatment intervention. The "Behavior Assessment System for Children" (BASC; Reynolds and Kamphaus, 1992) was used for pre and post measures. Parents completed the children-parent rating version (BASC-PRS); teachers completed the children-teacher scale (BASC-TRS), and the children completed the self-report (BASC-SRP).

The group sandtray therapists followed the Homeyer and Sweeney (1998) guidelines including the six-step session protocol: (1) room preparation, (2) introduction to the participant, (3) creation of the sand tray, (4) postcreation, (5) sand tray cleanup, and (6) documenting the session. The group members were instructed to look at the miniatures, use as many or few as they liked, and select a few that interested them. After placing them in the tray, they could add as many as they liked to "create a world in the sand." The sandtray therapist indicated she would sit quietly until they were finished. Thirty minutes of the 45-minute session were allotted for creation of the trays. The final 15 minutes were available for those group members who desired to share the story of their tray. The therapist asked a few facilitative questions as they shared the story of the tray. At the end of the group session, the trays were left intact. The therapist took pictures and documented the trays using one of the session forms found in Homeyer and Sweeney (1998) and added notes about any significant group interaction during the session.

Based on teachers' reports, there was a significant difference between the experimental and control groups, of $d = .52$ effect size in the total problem behavior score. This difference was reflective of the slight improvement of the sandtray therapy group, with the control group experiencing a worsening of behavior. In this same area, parents' reports of behavior showed no significant difference. Teachers' reports revealed a significant change in internalizing behavior between groups, $d = .59$, while parents did not. Both parents and teachers reported significant changes between groups in the area of externalizing behavior, $d = .54$ and $d = .63$, respectively. This research indicated that medium effect sizes were found in the above noted areas. It indicates that the sandtray therapy groups may have improved only slightly, but the behavior of the preadolescents in the control group continued to deteriorate during the time of the study. This finding supports the view that untreated problem behavior and mental health issues continue to worsen over time.

Shen (2006, Shen & Armstrong, 2008) used group sandtray therapy to study changes in the self-esteem of 37 seventh-grade adolescent girls. Using a pretest-posttest control group design, participants were assigned to groups based on pretest score means. This was done so group means would be equal. The Self-Perception Profile for Children (Harter, 1985) was used to collect pre and post data.

The experiential group was further divided into five groups of four girls each. Each group met for nine, 50-minute sessions twice a week for 4.5 weeks. Each girl built in a 21-inch round sand tray painted blue inside. The girls were allotted 15 minutes to build a scene, leaving 35 minutes to process the scene. The group sandtray therapist facilitated the processing with questions and used group skills to normalize and promote universality. The groups also were focused each session on a specific topic important to young adolescent girls, such as relationships, social acceptance, and physical appearance.

Based on the analysis of the data (Split-Plot Analysis of Variance, SPANOVA) the girls in the sandtray therapy group improved in the self-esteem areas of scholastic competence ($d = .68$), physical appearance ($d = .52$), global self-worth ($d = .83$), and behavioral conduct ($d = .64$) and showed possibilities of effectiveness in the area of social acceptance ($d = .46$).

Draper, Ritter and Willingham (2003) also researched sandtray group counseling with adolescents. The purpose of their study was "to help participants address intrapersonal concerns, learn important skills of socialization, and develop a caring community" (p. 244). The study occurred at an alternative school for middle and high school students. These students attended the alternative school because of disruptive behavioral problems and rule infractions. All 200 students attending the alternative school were offered the experience. Forty students returned parent permission forms and agreed to participate. Twenty-six students completed the group experience, which met for weekly sessions for 8 weeks. The students were separated into seven groups based on whether they were in middle or high school and by gender. There were some mixed gender groups because there were insufficient numbers of girls to constitute a group. The 1-hour session was divided into 25 minutes for building the scene, 5 minutes to take pictures, and the remaining 30 minutes to share the story and process the trays. Students were allowed to pass if they chose not to talk about their trays. The therapist modeled empathic, active listening with a summary reflection.

The researchers had the following descriptive comments regarding the dynamics of these sandtray groups. They found that these students were more likely to increase their willingness to express vulnerability, let their guard down, and be more authentic. Group members were quite cooperative regarding the selection of miniatures, a change from their typical competitive, aggressive interactions (p. 257). Groups varied on their interactions during the building phase. Some were quiet while others talked about important issues; other groups only discussed superficial topics. The sharing phase revealed members being very supportive of each other and a caring community was created.

In summary, Hughes (2004) effectively states the process of the group sandtray therapy:

> Metacognitive perception, knowledge about our own thoughts and the factors that influence our thinking, occurs in multiplicity around the group sand tray; each person considers her/his own assumptions in light of the others' perspectives. The activity presents a chance to practice openness, enhance understanding by listening to each other, adjust attitudes, develop positive traits, improve behavior towards each other and become a well-functioning whole. (p. 8)

A qualitative inquiry by Swank and Lenes (2013) looked at 20 adolescent girls, 12–17.6 years of age, attending an alternative school. Each group consisted of four adolescents, each working in her individual tray for weekly, 50-minute sessions, for a total of 5 weeks. They used a non-directive approach and were instructed to create their world/life in the sand (p. 336). Data were collected from semi-structured interview and focus groups and analyzed using a phenomenological method. They found five themes: self-expression, development of insight, growth opportunities, hope, and connecting through group dynamics. They also indicated the sand tray experience resulted found the girls "engaged in problem solving and healthy coping skills" (p. 344).

Bonds (1995) studied at-risk, inner-city Latino and African American adolescents (aged 16–20 years old) also attending an alternative high school. All subjects had previously dropped out of school. Bonds sought to see if sandtray therapy could be effective as a way to work with these difficult populations. Data were collected from 15 African American and 15 Latino adolescents' initial sand tray constructions and interviews. Each student was provided the choice to use a dry or wet rectangular tray and to select from a collection of approximately 600 miniatures. The prompt was very general: "Create anything you want . . . take all the time you want. I'll take two pictures when you are done" (p. 38).

A content analysis was conducted to identify similarities and differences between the two racial groups. Two-way ANOVAs analyzed the number and types of miniatures used, time to build the tray, and personal enjoyment of the building process. Girls and Latinos used significantly more animals. Significant use of aggressive human figures or objects was demonstrated by boys, but Latinas showed no use of aggressive items. Both groups identified the experience as very enjoyable. Of the participants, 100% of the girls and 90% of the boys indicated they would like to do another tray. While both groups used a high number of like-race people miniatures, they used other-race people as well, with no statistical significance.

In China, university students were studied by Wen, Risheng, Haslam and Zhiling (2011). Wen et al. studied nine students with serious social difficulties as identified by pre-intervention scores on the Social Avoidance and Distress Scale (SAD). A larger group sand tray of 22.5 inches by 28.5 inches by 2.75 inches (57 cm by 72 cm by 7 cm) provided room for all nine students to build together. Restricted Group Sandplay Therapy (RGST), developed by Risheng, was used in this study. Each member of the group rotated adding or moving/repositioning a miniature on each of their turns. A time for group discussion followed. The group completed eight sessions. The post-data collected with SAD showed a 60% positive change in pre-post mean scores for all nine of the students, indicating noticeable improvement.

SANDTRAY THERAPY TO IMPROVE CLASSROOM BEHAVIOR

Zarzaur (2004) studied teachers' perceptions of the improvement of behavior of students from kindergarten to fourth grade. This was a pretest-posttest control group design. Participants, in kindergarten to fourth grade, were referred by teachers, staff, school counselors, or self-referred. They were randomly assigned to receive either sandtray play therapy ($n = 13$) or classroom behavior management ($n = 13$). Pre- and posttreatment data was collected using the Achenbach Child Behavior Checklist (CBC, Achenbach, 1991) completed by homeroom teachers.

The students in the two treatment groups met for five, 30-minute, weekly individual sessions. The first session for all students was an intake session during which the counselor and student decided on an issue upon which to work. The remaining four sandtray therapy sessions followed the Homeyer and Sweeney (1998) six-step session protocol. A nondirective prompt was given allowing the student to "create your world in the sand." During the building phase, the counselor verbally tracked the student as one does in play therapy. Fifteen to 20 minutes were given to build the tray, with the remaining 10 to 15 minutes to process the tray. The students in the classroom behavior management group also had four individual sessions with the counselor and used contingency contracting as described by Thompson and Rudolph (2000). This included developing mutually acceptable goals, behavior contract to meet those goals, and discussion of progress toward those goals. Meeting the goals earned the student a reward and not meeting the goal resulted in loss of a privilege.

The data were analyzed using a repeated measure analysis of variance (ANOVA). The results indicated there were no statistically significant differences between or within groups on adaptive behavior scores. The sandtray therapy and classroom management group means for adaptive behavior, which the teachers rated on the CBC, were in the normal range before (3.05 and 3.67, respectively) and after (3.46 and 3.96) treatment. This indicates the homeroom teachers did see problem behaviors in the students, thus the referrals, but adaptive behavior was scored in the normal range both pretest and posttest.

There was, however, marked improvement in specific problem behaviors in pre and post data in the total score on the CBC. The teachers indicated behavioral symptoms decreased for both groups. The sandtray therapy and classroom management groups' total score means were in the clinical range before treatment (64.15 and 61.23, respectively). The posttest group means show the sandtray therapy group in the borderline ranges (61.92) and the classroom management group in the normal range (59.00). The same results were found regardless of gender.

Zarzaur (2004) indicates that because schools often use behavioral management techniques because of efficacy, this indicates that the sandtray therapy group could be as effective. Also, given that the sandtray therapy intervention used less school counselor and classroom teacher time, it could become the intervention of choice.

SANDTRAY THERAPY FOR VARIOUS PRESENTING PROBLEMS AND TREATMENT ISSUES

Couples Sandtray Therapy

Mason (1986) studied marital satisfaction and its relationship between individuality and mutuality. This repeated measures design collected data through observation and self-report, using both questionnaires and written stories of the trays. Eight couples were recruited from graduate-level communications and psychology classes. Four couples indicated considerable marital distress, the other four were non-distressed. The couples had been married for an average of 2 years (range of 6 months to 4 years). The mean age for the men was 34 and 30 for the women. Over a period of 3 months, the couples began with building an individual tray. Then three couples' trays were constructed. The experience ended with a final individual tray. The couples' trays included the dynamics of what to decide to build, what to include, how to negotiate differences, and whether to divide or share the territory. The sand tray creations were scored on a researcher-developed, literature-based system. The ratings included: lifeless/populated, aggressive/peaceful, empty/full, rigid/chaotic, stereotypes/unique, guarded/open, overall feeling tone of positive/negative, and space sharing. The interviews were coded for couple-oriented problem solving, individual approach to problem solving, agreement, disagreement, humor, aggression, reach for understanding, feeling talk, and metacommunication. Qualitative analyses revealed that non-distressed couples developed a storyline in their shared sand tray building over time. Non-distressed spouses also emphasized their coupleness in both their individual and couple sand trays, and were able to feel closer and more separate than their unhappy counterparts. Distressed couples expressed problems connected with being together and with being apart, and disagreed on how much closeness or distance was optimal.

Adult Sandtray Therapy

No and Kim (2013) studied eight university students in Korea with ADHD tendencies. The students participated in individual, weekly sessions for 10 weeks. The data was analyzed using the Wilcoxon Signed Rank Test. This study found there were significant differences in terms of decreases in anxiety, interpersonal stress, and salivary cortisol. It also suggests that sandplay therapy has significantly positive effects on the anxiety, interpersonal stress, and salivary cortisol levels of students with ADHD tendencies who are experiencing pressures and conflicts in university life.

Adult male substance abuse offenders in an inpatient facility participated in a qualitative, phenomenological study on their perceptions of Adlerian sandtray therapy as an adjunct to cognitive behavioral rehabilitative treatment (Monakes, Garza, Weisner, & Watts, 2011). The four participants, ranging in age from 22–40 years, participated in five individual sandtray therapy sessions. Each session was focused on Adlerian concepts: 1) Identifying information, prompt: "Create a tray of one of your earliest memories"; 2) Presenting information, prompt: "What brings you here and why now?"; 3) Current functioning on life tasks, prompt: "How has the presenting problem affected or not affected you in these areas?"; 4) Work, social life and love; Goals of treatment, prompt: "What would be different in your life if you didn't have this particular problem?"; and, 5) Treatment expectations, prompt: "What is keeping you from your goal and what would you like to do about it?" (p. 99). Each session began with 15 minutes to build the scene followed by time to process the tray, following the Homeyer and Sweeney (1998) guidelines. A sixth session was an unstructured interview, reviewing the five sand trays and the participants' perceptions of the experience.

Using Colaizzi's phenomenological analysis, Monakes et al. identified the following themes: It was a positive experience (had fun, wished for more such experiences, and found it helpful); insight provoking (with the opportunity to be reflective, sobering self-reflection, and heightening awareness of the relationship between past and current experiences), helping with goal setting (ability to reevaluate, make plans, and improve self-efficacy); discovering a new form of self-expression (through the interaction with their material in the tray creating meaning and experience of going deeper); and, initially experienced as unpleasant (based in the fear of being judged, unsure of the process and what happens with the outcome). Finally, in the comparison of adding sandtray therapy to the regularly offered treatment, the four participants indicated the sand tray therapy atmosphere resulted in higher levels of trust, and appreciation for the individualized interaction compared to the regular center's basic atmosphere which was sensed as not exploring sufficiently deep, insincere, and not personalized) (p. 102). The researchers believe the use of sandtray therapy facilitates the connection with the offender and mental health professionals.

Adolescent Sandtray Therapy

Artico (2000) studied the perceptions and memories of Latino adolescents separated in childhood and later reunited with their parents because of piecemeal immigration patterns. This research can provide insight to professionals working with Latino, and perhaps other immigrants, to assist these families to integrate this experience and rebuild broken relationships. Three male and four female Latino adolescents, ages 15 to 19, participated in the in-depth interviews and sand tray activity.

Artico used a topical design to focus on the issue of separation from parents and ways it affected the relationship with self and others (p. 194). The computer program, *N-Vivo* (1994), was used to code interviews, resulting in 30 categories. The sand trays were mapped using the eight basic configurations developed by Ryce-Menuhin (1992). These configurations provide the therapist with possible insights into the meaning of the tray and its builder. Sand trays were also evaluated for relevant elements of construction and content analysis according to the Erica Method of Assessment (Sjolund & Schaefer, 1994). The sand trays revealed anxiety, depression, and regrets about relocating to the United States. Differences were found between trays of those who were less distressed about life and relationships with caretakers and parents and those with more disturbed affect and adjustment difficulties (p. 207). Interviews resulted in categories such as abandonment, sacrifice, divided loyalties, role reversal, losses, guilt, shame, damaged goods, and heroes. Implications for mental health practitioners include to facilitate more open, frequent, accepting, and empathic communication; avoid competition with and criticism of previous caretakers; awareness of the impact of the continuity vs. discontinuity of care; identifying the behaviors of unconditional love and finally, to provide opportunities for education regarding these dynamics and referrals for interventions for these children who are often at higher risk because of disrupted attachments.

Child Sandtray Therapy

Separation anxiety of 5–7-year-olds in Tehran was studied by Nasab and Alipour (2015) using a quasi-experimental pretest-posttest control group design. Thirty children (15 boys and 15 girls), diagnosed with separation anxiety, were randomly assigned into the experiential and control groups. Children in the experiential group received ten, 1-hour sessions which followed the Lowenfeld sand tray model (p. 7). Lowenfeld's model, as reported by Nasab and Alipour, has goals for each of the ten sessions although no details were given on how these goals were implemented. Analyzing data collected with the Child Symptom Inventory-4 resulted in between-group factor finding significance at level 0.01 ($p = 0.01$, $F(1.26) = (63.7)$) (p. 9). No details were provided on the procedures within the sand tray sessions. Given the findings, the researchers recommend that all kindergartens in the country work with mental health centers to treat children with separation anxiety.

Immigrant and refugee families may have significant mental health issues based in the trauma of persecution and organized violence before the migration. The trauma can be exacerbated by subsequent observation of media exposure to a catastrophe of their home of origin or natural disaster. Schools who serve these populations provide experiences to remediate with a variety of cultural and other experiences. Rousseau, Benoit, Lacroix and Gauthier (2009) did an evaluative study of 105 primarily South Asian kindergartners who resided in multi-ethnic neighborhoods. The children were randomly assigned and participated in ten 60-minute sandplay sessions held every other week. The sand tray time was built into the regular school day schedule and led by art therapists. Two children built in one tray which had a removable divider. The set of miniature figures had additional culturally diverse items such as deities of several religions, flags of different countries, diverse national costumes. Each session had three parts: 1) Opening ritual of circle time, singing an action song; 2) Creating in the sand tray (time to build, then telling their stories); 3) closing ritual of and other circle time and singing an action song. Pretest and posttest data were collected with the Strengths and Differences Questionnaire completed by teachers and parents. Analysis of the data showed statistically significant at $p = 0.001$. Rousseau et al. concluded that sandplay sessions can provide children the opportunity to work though feelings of fears and worries subsequent to being exposed to natural disasters and human-made traumatic events while also being preventive to retriggering trauma responses (p. 749).

Sandplay as an intervention for a 7-year-old boy with autism was selected by Parker and O'Brien (2011) because it is a form of play therapy with a high sensory stimulation (p. 82). Parker and O'Brien added soft music playing in the background for additional stimulation. Using a case study research design, the boy was selected using information-oriented sampling. He had been referred to the school guidance officer (Australia) because of his high number of classroom tantrums, hitting and biting of other children in the playground, and refusal to participate in classroom activities (p. 83). Other interventions had been unsuccessful. The number of incidents of these behaviors was noted daily over 12 weeks of sandplay treatment which consisted of 12, 45-minute sessions. After the completion of the intervention the number of problems behaviors dropped sharply. The total behavior declined from over 35 incidents per week to fewer than five; the other four identified problem behaviors also dropped to under five per week. His refusal to participate in class and classroom tantrums, were eliminated (p. 85). Parker and O'Brien suggest that given the verbal and social interaction deficits of children with autism, sandplay, as a form of play therapy, may offer additional alternatives for counseling these children (p. 86).

Depression in young adolescents, ages 11–14, was studied by Dawson (2011). She used a multiple-baseline-across-participants single-case design. Four young adolescents and their mothers completed questionnaires throughout the process, beginning with a baseline, then as treatment occurred. The young adolescents completed a four-item depression symptom questionnaire daily during base-line data collection; and prior to their weekly sand tray therapy sessions. Intervention was one session a week for 12–14 weeks. The sessions were held in a private practice office, with one sand tray and several shelves of miniature objects organized by category. The initial prompt as "make a world in the sand" (p. 65), although two participants asked for further clarification. After the building was complete, the researcher asked: "Can you tell me as much or as little as you want to about your world?", "Where would you be in this world?", and "Can you give your world a title?" (p. 66). Dawson found that three of the four participants showed improvement in their depression symptoms, showing "credence to the efficacy of sand tray therapy in treatment of depression in young people" (p. 126). Additionally, she related that use of the sand tray assisted in the development of building trust and the working alliance; it also allowed the therapy process to be deeper and richer (p. 132).

Plotkin (2011) studied the effects of parental divorce on children. Her experiential pretest-posttest group design studied 32, 6- to 10-year-old children who had experienced divorce within the past 2 years. The 16 children in the experiential group each participated in eight sessions of 'sandtray play therapy' defined by Plotkin as: "a multidimensional form of play therapy that utilizes a tray partially filled with sand and a large collection of miniature figures" (p. 11). The other 16 children were in a wait-list control group. The Child Behavior Checklist was used pre and post to collect data on internalizing and externalizing behavior. The researcher conducting the eight, 30-minute individual sandtray play therapy sessions was a mental health professional with 36 hours of additional training in sandtray play therapy, and 4 years' experience using this modality. The children were informed they could use as many or as few figures as they wanted, when the building was completed, the tray was discussed. The findings show statistically significant (set at 0.05) differences between the experiential and control group on both internalizing (p= 0.021) and externalizing (p= 0.043) behavior. There were no differences between genders (p. 64–71).

Sandtray construction was used as one of several assessment methods to identify resilience in children affected by war. Fernando (2006) studied what promoted adaptive or maladaptive development of the children of war in Sri Lanka. The study involved 62 orphaned children and 15 caregivers. Children ranged between 5 and 18 years of age and caregivers were between 25 to 80 years of age. Fernando used the sandtray to primarily assess for internalizing difficulties and emotional reactions. The Sandtray World View Scale developed by Jones (1986) provided a second look at cognitive development. This did result in identifying two children as below age level in cognitive development. These two children were also identified at the highest risk, given their life experience as war orphans. They had witnessed raids on their villages, killings, and separation from their families. The cognitive levels identified in the sandtrays were generally supported by the results of the Goodenough-Harris Drawings. The sandtray constructions and narratives were also analyzed according to Kurt Fischer's Structural Analyses (Fischer & Bidell, 2006). This revealed that conceptual complexities of stories and narratives increased with age. Clinical perspectives of the sandtray stories revealed significant differences between nonproblematic, nonproblematic with war content, and potential clinical concern relating to war (p. 114). Chi-square analysis of the differences between the three groups was significant at $p < .002$. Data revealed 50% of the war orphans' sandtray worlds had "themes of war experiences, death, poverty, loss and abandonment" and the trays were identified as having stories of clinical concern (p. 115). The children identified as having clinical concerns, however, were also identified as competent in areas of academic motivation, peer relationships, and social conduct (p. 118).

Howell (1999) investigated the influence of children's cognitive ability and level of bereavement on their perceptions of death and danger. Sixty 5- to 12-year-old children (mean age, 8 years 4 months) participated in the study with thirty children each in the bereaved group and nonbereaved groups. The children in the bereaved group experienced the death of a close loved one in the past 5 years. A sandtray experience was one of several measures for this study. A sandtray measure was specifically designed and validated for this study. This included Indexes of Danger and Death, Death Preoccupation, and Defensiveness. The children were given a nondirected prompt, which in part was to simply "make a picture in the sand." Using a Chi-square analysis, no significant differences were found between the two groups on the Index of Death Preoccupation ($p = 0.43$) or on the Index of Defensiveness ($p = 0.50$). A significant difference ($p = 0.03$) was found on the Index of Danger and Death. The bereaved group had 64% of the children who displayed indicators of danger and death, while only 37% of the nonbereaved group did so. An interesting finding was that children in both groups spontaneously placed symbols and had play themes of death in their sandtrays (53% in nonbereaved, 43% in bereaved). While comparing all children, the boys displayed significantly more indicators of preoccupation with death and danger than the girls. This may be because boys showed more aggressive themes, one of the scored items for indicators for death and danger. This is consistent with other studies of boys play in the sandtray.

RESEARCH OF OTHER USES OF SAND TRAY

Clinical Supervision in Graduate Programs

The use of the sand tray in supervision of master's level counseling students was studied by Stark, Garza, Bruhn and Ane (2015). Using a convenience sample of five students already together for a clinical practicum experience at the university's community clinic, the five female students (32–50 age range) participated in three sand tray experiences during their semester of supervised clinical work. Given all these student-supervisees had the school counseling specialty and that the solution-focused approach often used in school settings, the supervisor used a solution-focused supervision approach as well. The supervisor was a counselor educator who is a registered play therapist and had advanced training in both sandtray therapy and the solution-focused approach. The prompt for the first sandtray supervision session was to create a scene of "what was improving in their counseling"; second session included fast-forwarding questions (e.g., "what will take place 3 weeks in the future?"), relationship questions (e.g., "what will your classmates observe in your counseling?"), and goal setting. The last session included asking the supervisees to use the miniatures to symbolize varying levels of success, in a way that would anchor their scaling (p. 6). Qualitative data were collected using the participant's reflective journals of each sand tray experience and interviews after the final session. Constructivist research analysis of the interviews found two major themes: (a) participant learning was aided by experiencing the blended approach, and (b) the supervision approach with the sand tray was found to be helpful on a personal level. The analysis of the journals found the primary of emotionality (e.g., processing their own emotions regarding stressful co-existing events) and group cohesiveness (e.g., peer support and positive feedback of the emotionally stressful disclosures; p. 8–9). Stark et al. believe the addition of the sandtray experiences assisted in the personal development of the supervisees, an important component of clinical development.

Pilot study research comparing the effectiveness of adding sand tray experiences to supervision with traditional supervision (didactic self-report and case presentations) was conducted by Markos, Coker and Jones (2008). The six female participants ranged in age from 24–50 years old and were in two convenient sample groups (one marriage and family focused, the other school counseling focused), during their required practicum courses. Data were collected using the Supervisory Working Alliance Inventory (Efstation, Patton, & Kardash, 1990) which the participants of both groups completed after each weekly supervision session. Both groups used the traditional method of supervision in the first half of the semester; then 4 weeks of sandtray experiences were added.

In the sandtray experiences group, for example, the researchers used the prompt: *"Focus on this client. Now put your client's situation in the sand."* And then added, *"Put yourself as counselor in the sand related to the case."* Although the supervision sessions when students utilized the sand tray resulted in higher (more positive) responses in both the Rapport and Client Focus subscales of the analysis pre-post scores, no statistical significance was found. However, observationally, the researchers reported an increased ability to "kinesthetically and visually represent their client's concerns and contexts, and establish a vision for change" (p. 12; Homeyer, in press).

Sandtray in Multicultural Counselor Training in Graduate Programs

Based on the understanding that the use of sand tray facilitates self-awareness and unconscious issues, Paone, Malott, Gao and Kinda (2015) explored how the use of sandplay in a race-based multicultural counseling course would assist students in the same areas. Using a qualitative, phenomenological inquiry approach, Paone et al. studied 43 master-level counseling students, ages 21–37 years-old. The racial make-up of the students was white (88%), Latino (7%), and multiracial (5%); 86% were female, 14% were male (p. 193). The four authors were White (2), Black (1) and Asian (1). The lead researcher was a counselor educator and a registered play therapy-supervisor. The participants attended one of five multicultural courses. During their course they created three sandtrays, at the beginning, middle, and end of a typical 15-week semester. Each student worked in a small tray, 12″ by 9.75″ and 3″ filled with 1.5″ of sand. They collectively used a set of 200 miniatures (with additional various miniature figures of various races and age groups) placed on the floor in the middle of the group. The prompt to the students was to create their journey so far in the course, including where they are developmentally and to express feelings and perceptions regarding the course (p. 194). After the sandtray creation was completed the students shared their trays with their peers. Data was collected using student journals (written after each sandtray experience), photograph of the tray, written reposes to questions regarding the sandplay, and a final focus group (transcribed for analysis). Analysis found the following: Second order themes with corresponding first order themes:

1. Sandtray as a positive experience; enjoyable and beneficial;
2. Sandtray facilitated new learning; unconscious became conscious; increased self-understanding;
3. Sandtray meaningful in a group context; seeing others' sandtrays facilitated connection, reduced own negative affect;
4. Sandtray facilitated expression; emotional expression, visual expression;
5. Difficulties with sandtray; initial difficulties, mismatch of learning styles (p. 204).

The researchers concluded that the use of the sand tray experience facilitated the students' development of greater insight into their racial identify growth (p. 201).

CONCLUSION

The increase of research in sandtray therapy is very encouraging. More quantitative studies on the efficacy of sand tray therapy in particular is growing. We encourage researchers to be diligent in clearly identifying the population, the specific treatment and methodology, and the qualifications of the researchers. It is particularly important to identify the theoretical approach to the utilization of sandtray therapy. Like play therapy, sandtray therapy is a generic term for many applications and approaches. It would be helpful for those reading the research to know if the researcher used Adlerian, Child-Centered, Gestalt, Cognitive-Behavioral, Solution Focused, etc. applications in the research study. These all are quite varied and having more specifics on the protocol would assist the reader in applying the findings to their own clinical work.

Additionally, there are several dissertations which have not yet been published in professional journals. We encourage graduates in doing so. We are well aware of the exhaust-factor which comes after completing the dissertation. However, many of them have valuable findings which would benefit the field at large, in a more easily assess-able way.

Finally, we encourage current and future researchers to replicate studies in the ongoing quest to establish sandtray therapy as an evidence-based treatment. We are building a solid collection of empirical-based studies. It's a great initial step and we thank every researcher who has added to our growing body of sandtray therapy literature.

Appendix A: Session Notes and Other Forms

Organizing the content and details of a sandtray therapy session varies from play therapy to adult, talk therapy. We have both developed forms on which to document a session. We invite you, the reader, to feel free to copy either of these forms for your own use. Or, feel free to use some of the ideas on the forms and adapt for your own use.

SANDTRAY THERAPY SESSION SUMMARIES

Both forms are in the format to quickly circle, underline, or check items. Aware of the short amount of time between sessions, this is helpful for quick documentation, then at a later time, to return and provide narrative.

These versions no longer have the 'box' to draw the sand tray creation. If you prefer to draw, please use the back. We have found almost everyone is taking a digital figure which is printed out then stapled as a second page. In the top right corner is a place to indicate by circling a Yes or a No, if a photo was taken. This can be a reminder to print out and attach.

SANDTRAY THERAPY INFORMED CONSENTS AND CONSENT FOR TRAINING AND/OR PUBLISHING

Additionally, we have noticed in the training and supervision of counselors, play therapists, and sandtray therapists, that too few use appropriate informed consent forms or specific consent forms to use sandtray pictures for training and educational purposes. We have included a sample of each for sandtray therapists to consider for use in their practice.

SELF-EVALUATION FORM

The self-evaluation form is useful to assist the sandtray therapist in assessing a session and for skill development. This can also be used by supervisors to provide feedback to supervisees.

Any of these may also be photocopied or adapted for your own use.

SANDTRAY THERAPY SESSION SUMMARY

Date: _____   Session # _____   Photo: Yes   No

Client's Name _____

I. CLIENT APPROACH: Underline all that apply

Ease / Difficult—getting started   Able / Unable to be fully engaged   Use of Miniatures: Use of Time: All / Part
Determined / Hesitant   Internally / Externally driven   Avoided: Use of Space: All / Part
Purposeful / Non-purposeful   Verbal / Non-verbal   Held /Caressed: Use of Water: Yes / No
Other: Placed, then removed: Number of Scenes: _____

II: OBJECTIVE: Underline all that apply

A. Sandtray Organization:

Empty . . . . Excessive
Open . . . . Closed/Fenced
Action . . . . Static
One Idea . . . . . Several Ideas
Rigid . . . . Realistic
Organized . . . . Disorganized/Chaotic
Unpeopled . . . . People

B. Miniatures Used:

People: _____

Animals: _____

Vegetation: _____

Buildings: _____

Fences/Signs: _____

Cartoon/Movie: _____

Fantasy/Spiritual: _____

Household Items: _____

Landsacaping/Natural: _____

Other: _____

C. Significant Verbalization during Building Scene:

III. ASSESSMENT: General Impressions / Clinical Understanding

A. Themes: Underline all that apply; describe how theme was shown through miniatures & arrangement. Circle predominate theme.
   Conflict / Violence:
   Aggression / Anger / Revenge:
   Death / Loss / Grieving / Abandonment:
   Secretive / Buried:
   Power / Control:
   Helpless / Inadequate:
   Empty / Depressed:
   Safety / Security / Protection:
   Relationships:
   Spiritual:
   Other:

B. Prompt

_____

C. Discussion of Tray
Title:

_____

D. Conceptualization of Client and Client's Progress:

IV. PLANS / RECOMMENDATIONS:

Counselor: _____   Date: _____

SANDTRAY WORKSHEET

Date: _____   Session # _____   Photo: Yes   No

Client's Name: _____

Prompt: _____

Title of the tray: _____ Wet: Yes   No   Dry _____

Description of the tray: _____ organized _____ chaotic _____ peaceful _____ aggressive _____ violent _____ depressed
                                              _____ healing/helpful _____ open _____ closed _____ secretive/buried
                                              _____ other (describe_____)

Miniature figures chosen:

   People: _____

   Animals: _____

   Vegetation: _____

   Buildings: _____

   Fences/Signs: _____

   Cartoon/Movie: _____

   Fantasy/Spiritual: _____

   Household Items: _____

   Landsacaping/Natural: _____

   Other: _____

Describe client's verbal and affective expressions during tray construction:

_____
_____
_____
_____

Describe the story (metaphors/themes) about the tray offered by the client:

_____
_____
_____
_____

Summarize discussion of tray:

_____
_____
_____
_____

Conceptualization of process:

_____
_____
_____
_____

Plan/Referral:

_____
_____
_____
_____

Counselor: _____ Date: _____

SAMPLE CONSENT FOR SANDTRAY THERAPY

I affirm that prior to becoming a client, I was given sufficient information to understand the nature of counseling and sandtray therapy. This information included, but was not limited to, the nature of the counseling practice or agency, the professional identity and qualifications of the counselor, the possible risks and benefits of counseling, the nature of confidentiality including legal and ethical limits, and alternative treatments available. I have had all my questions answered fully.

I agree that I have sought and consent to take part in the sandtray therapy by the counselor named below. I understand the importance of the development of a treatment plan and the need to regularly review treatment goals. I agree to play an active role in this process. I further understand that no guarantees have been made to me as to the results of the counseling and sandtray process.

I understand that a photographic record will be kept of the sandtray therapy, and that these photographs will become part of the permanent client record, following all applicable legal and ethical rules of confidentiality.

I understand that any cancellation of an appointment must be made at least 24 hours before the time of the appointment. If I do not cancel or do not show up, I understand that I will be charged for that appointment.

My signature below affirms that I have read and understand and agree with the statements above, and that I voluntarily consent to counseling and sandtray therapy.

_____   _____

Signature of client   Date

Minor client: I affirm that I am the legal guardian of_____.
My signature below affirms that I have read and understand the statements above, and that I voluntarily consent to counseling and sandtray therapy for the child named above.

_____   _____

Signature of client   Date

_____   _____

Signature of client   Date

RELEASE AND PERMISSION TO VIDEOTAPE SESSIONS AND/OR PHOTOGRAPH SANDTRAYS FOR EDUCATIONAL PURPOSES

I would like to use your (or your child's) video-recorded and/or photographed material in teaching, supervision, consultation with other therapists, or publishing. I would like to have your written permission to make and use these recordings for these purposes. This includes:

■ Audio or video recordings of our sessions.
■ Photographs of sandtrays, drawings, or other art creations.

When I use materials from my therapy work, I do not want anyone who hears, reads, or sees it to be able to identify my client(s) involved. Therefore, I would conceal your (or your child's) identity by removing (or significantly changing) all names, dates, places, descriptions, or any other information by which you or anyone else involved could be identified.

These materials will be shown only to other mental health professionals and/or students. All of these persons are bound by state laws and professional rules about clients' privacy. I will keep all these materials in a safe location, and destroy them as soon as they are no longer needed.

_____

Therefore, I am asking you to read and sign the following:

I, the client (or his or her parent or guardian), consent to the video recording or photographs described above. The purpose and value of recording have been fully explained to me, and I freely and willingly consent to this recording.

This consent is being given for the therapist named below. I understand that there will not be any negative consequences if I do not wish a particular session or project to be recorded.

I give the therapist named below my permission to use the recordings for research, teaching, and other professional purposes. I understand that they will be used as an aid in the process of improving mental health work or training mental health workers. These professionals and their students are bound by state laws and by professional rules about clients' privacy.

I agree to let the therapist be the sole owner of all the rights in these recordings for all purposes described above.

_____
Printed name of client

_____   _____
Signature of client (or parent/guardian)   Date

_____
Printed name of therapist

_____   _____
Signature of therapist   Date

SELF-EVALUATION FORM: SANDTRAY THERAPY

		RANGE Needs work— Average—Excellent				COMMENTS

PROMPT

Gives Directions to Client

1.	Clear, concise	1	2	3	4	5	_____
2.	Intentional, appropriate	1	2	3	4	5	_____

CREATIVE

Observing the Process

3.	Empathic and present	1	2	3	4	5	_____
4.	Identifies approach to task	1	2	3	4	5	_____
5.	Identifies emotional expression	1	2	3	4	5	_____
6.	Identifies behavior	1	2	3	4	5	_____

PROCESSING

Use of creation (sandtray, art)

7.	Use of metaphor, image	1	2	3	4	5	_____
8.	Fully explores content of tray	1	2	3	4	5	_____

Immediacy

9.	Fosters specific verbalizations	1	2	3	4	5	_____
10.	Uses information from creation process	1	2	3	4	5	_____

Understands content and context

11.	Conveys accurate understanding	1	2	3	4	5	_____
12.	Reflects content	1	2	3	4	5	_____
13.	Clarifies	1	2	3	4	5	_____
14.	Summarizes	1	2	3	4	5	_____
15.	Reflects feeling	1	2	3	4	5	_____

Establishes and communicates empathy

16.	Communicates warmth, acceptance and respect	1	2	3	4	5	_____
17.	Constructive, genuine verbalizations	1	2	3	4	5	_____

Creates structure

18.	Able to initiate and terminate session	1	2	3	4	5	_____
19.	Manages time and allows for processing	1	2	3	4	5	_____

OVERALL COUNSELOR SKILLS

20.	Counselor looked comfortable	1	2	3	4	5	_____
21.	Appropriate eye contact	1	2	3	4	5	_____
22.	Paced session (including use of silence)	1	2	3	4	5	_____
23.	Voice consistent with client's message	1	2	3	4	5	_____
24.	Voice consistent with counselor's message	1	2	3	4	5	_____

Appendix B: Resources

MINIATURE FIGURES

Anna's Toy Depot
2620 S. Lamar Blvd #B
Austin, TX 78704
Phone: 1-888-227-9169
Fax: 1-512-447-4506
www.annastoydepot.com

Child Therapy Toys
3355 Bee Cave Road #610
Austin, TX 78746
Phone: 1-866-324-7529
Fax: 1-512-347-7189
E-mail: toys@childtherapytoys.com
www.childtherapytoys.com

Constructive Playthings
13201 Arrington Rd.
Grandview, Missouri 64030
Phone: 1-800-448-1412
Fax: 1-816-761-9295
Email: cp@constructiveplaythings.com
www.ustoyco.com or www.constructiveplaythings.com

The Feelings Company
30101 Town Center Drive, Suite 110
Laguna Niguel, CA 92677
Phone: 1-800-347-5017
Fax: 1-949-363-0206
E-mail: feelingscompany@cox.net
www.feelingscompany.com

Lakeshore Learning Materials
2695 E. Dominguez St.
Carson, CA 90895
Phone: 1-800-428-4414
Fax: 1-310-537-5403
www.lakeshorelearning.com

Play Therapy Supply Company
PO Box 7
Argos, IN 46501
Fax: 1-866-697-9994
Email: info@playtherapysupply.com
www.playtherapysupply.com

Self-Esteem Shop
32839 Woodward Ave Royal Oak, MI 48073
Phone: 1 (800) 251-8336 or 1 (248) 549-9900
email: selfesteemshop@gmail.com
Website: www.selfesteemshop.com

Toys of the Trade
838 E. High St. #289
Lexington, KY 40502
Phone: 1-866-461-2929
Fax: 1-866-803-3781
Email: toytrade@yahoo.com
www.toysofthetrade.com

SANDTRAY FURNITURE (TRAYS, SHELVES, AND CARTS)

Aspen Sand Trays
George Ridgeway and Jan Pacifico
PO Box 131
Tomé, NM 87060
Phone: 1-505-866-0582 orders / office
E-mail: potluck55@aol.com
www.aspensandtrays.com

Ron's Trays
Phone: 1-707-894-4856
E-mail: sandtrayman@gmail.com
www.sandtrays.com

Also See: (Details Previous Page)
Child Therapy Toys
Lakeshore Learning Materials
Self-Esteem Shop

Sand
Jurassic Sand
1961 Scenic Drive
Salt Lake City, UT 84108
Phone: 1-877-531-8600
www.jurassicsand.com
sandman@jurassicsand.com

Add Your Own Resources

Appendix C: Sand Tray Assessment Worksheet

This worksheet provides the user a single space to review and notate an assessment of a sand tray. It combines the normative data information and Bühler's clinical indicators as described in Chapter 11.

SAND TRAY ASSESSMENT WORKSHEET

Client: _____

Developmental Cognitive Stage
□ **Intuitive: 4–7** □ **Concrete: 8–12** □ **Formal: 12–Adult**

Use of Sand: _____

Boundaries

Sand use: _____

Figure grouping: _____

Boundary figures: _____

Anomalies disrupting/Odd placements:_____

Organization of Parts

Category of figures: _____

Orientation of figures: _____

Relationship between figures: _____

World View: _____

Theme

**Clinical Indicators
(Circle)**

Empty

   <5 categories/7 yrs. +

   <50 figures/8 yrs. +

   No human figures

Aggressive

   Soldiers fighting

   Animals biting

   Wild animals fighting

Distorted / 5 yrs. +

   Closed/fenced

   Disorganized

     Odd placements

     Disconnected

     Chaotic

   Rigid

     Schematic

     Rows

NOTES:

Appendix D: Selected Bibliography

We have found the following books to be helpful in learning about the sandtray therapy process. There are a wide variety of theoretical and technical approaches represented. We encourage the interested reader to select resources with which he/she personally and professionally resonates.

Allan, J. (1988). *Inscapes of the child's world: Jungian counseling in schools and clinics.* Dallas, TX: Spring Publications, Inc.

Ammann, R. (1991). *Healing and transformation in sandplay: Creative processes become visible.* La Salle, IL: Open Court Publishing Company.

Armstrong, S. (2009). *Sandtray therapy: A humanistic approach.* Dallas, TX: Lubic Press.

Boik, B. L., & Goodwin, E. A. (2000). *Sandplay therapy: A step-b-step manual for psychotherapists for diverse orientations.* New York, NY: Norton & Company.

Bradway, K. (1997). *Sandplay: Silent workshop of the psyche.* London: Routledge.

Bradway, K., Signell, K. A., Spare, G. H., Stewart, C. T., Stewart, L. H., & Thompson, C. (1981). *Sandplay studies: Origins, theory, and practice.* San Francisco, CA: C.G. Jung Institute.

Bradway, K., Signell, K. A., Spare, G. H., Stewart, C. T., Stewart, L. H., & Thompson, C. (1988). *Sandplay studies: Origins, theory and practice* (2nd ed.). Boston: Sigo Press.

Carey, L. J. (1999). *Sandplay therapy with children and families.* Northvale, NJ: Jason Aronson, Inc.

DeDomenico, G. S. (1995). *Sandtray world play: A comprehensive guide to the use of the sandtray in psychotherapeutic and transformational settings.* Oakland, CA: Vision Quest Images.

Dundas, E. T. (1978). *Symbols come alive in the sand.* Aptos, CA: Aptos Press.

Gil, E. (1994). *Play in family therapy.* New York: Guilford Press.

Green, E. (2014). *The handbook of Jungian play therapy with children and adolescents.* Baltimore, MD: John Hopkins University Press.

Hunter, L. (1998). *Images of resiliency: Troubled children create healing stories in the language of the sandplay.* Palm Beach, FL: Behavioral Communications Institute.

Kalff, D. (1980). *Sandplay: A psychotherapeutic approach to the psyche.* Santa Monica, CA: Sigo Press.

Landreth, G., Sweeney, D., Ray, D., Homeyer, L., & Glover, G. (2005). *Play therapy interventions with children's problems* (2nd ed.). Northvale, NJ: Jason Aronson, Inc.

Lowenfeld, M. (1967). *Play in childhood.* New York: John Wiley & Sons.

Lowenfeld, M. (1979). *The world technique.* London: Allen & Unwin.

Mattson, D., & Veldorale-Brogan, A. (2010). Objectifying the sand tray: An initial example of three-dimensional art image analysis for assessment. *The Arts in Psychotherapy, 37,* 90–96.

Mitchell, R. R., & Friedman, H. S. (1994). *Sandplay: Past, present and future.* London: Routledge.

Oaklander, V. (1978). *Windows to our children.* Moab, UT: Real People Press.

Piaget, J. (1969). *The theory of stages in cognitive development.* New York: McGraw-Hill.

Rogers, C. (1951). *Client-centered theory.* Boston, MA: Houshton Mifflin.

Ryce-Menuhin, J. (1991). *Jungian sandplay: The wonderful therapy.* London: Routledge.

Sweeney, D., & Homeyer, L. (1999). *Handbook of group play therapy.* San Francisco: Jossey-Bass, Inc. Publishers.

Sweeney, D., Baggerly, J., & Ray, D. (2014). *Group play therapy: A dynamic approach.* New York: Routledge Publishers.

Turner, B. (2005). *The handbook of sandplay therapy.* Cloverdale, CA: Temenos Press.

Turner, B. (in press). *The Routledge international handbook of sandplay therapy.* England: Routledge.

Unnsteinsdottir, K., & Turner, B. (2015). *Sandtray play in education: A teacher's guide.* Cloverdale, CA: Temenos Press.

Weinrib, E. L. (1983). *Images of the self: The sandplay therapy process.* Boston: Sigo Press.

Wells, H. G. (1911). *Floor games.* New York: Arno Press.

Wernar, C. (1956). *The effects of motor handicap on personality.* III. Child Development, *27,* 1.

Zunni, V. R. (1997). Differential aspects of sandplay with 10– and 11-year-old children. *Child Abuse & Neglect, 21*(7), 657–668.

References

Achenbach, T. M. (1991). *Manual for the teacher's report*. Burlington, VT: Department of Psychiatry, University of Vermont.

Ackerman, N. (1970). Child participation in family therapy. *Family Process, 9*(4), 403–410.

Allan, J. (1988). *Inscapes of the child's world: Jungian counseling in schools and clinics*. Dallas, TX: Spring Publications, Inc.

Allan, J. (2007, July). Jungian play therapy. Paper presented at the Play Therapy Summer Institute, Center for Play Therapy, University of North Texas, Denton, Texas.

American Psychiatric Association. (2013). *Diagnostic and statistical manual of mental disorders: DSM-5*. Washington, DC: American Psychiatric Association.

Anekstein, A., Hoskins, W., Astramovich, R., Garner, D., & Terry, J. (2014). 'Sandtray supervision': Integrating supervision models and sandtray therapy. *Journal of Creativity in Mental Health, 9*(1), 122–134.

Artico, C. I. (2000). Perceptions and memories of Latino adolescents separated in childhood due to piecemeal patterns of immigration. (Doctoral dissertation, Fairfax, VA: George Mason University). *Dissertation Abstract International*, AAT 9985096.

Badenoch, B. (2008). *Being a brain-wise therapist: A practical guide to interpersonal neurobiology*. New York: W.W. Norton & Company.

Badenoch, B., & Kestly, T. (2015). Exploring the neuroscience of healing play at every age. In D. Crenshaw & A. Stewart (Eds.), *Play therapy: A comprehensive guide to theory and practice* (pp. 524–538). New York: Guilford Press.

Beck, A., & Weishaar, M. (2005). Cognitive therapy. In R. Corsini & D. Wedding (Eds.), *Current psychotherapies* (7th ed.), (pp. 238–268). Belmont, CA: Thomson.

Bertoia, J. (1999). The invisible village: Jungian group play therapy. In D. Sweeney & L. Homeyer (Eds.), *The handbook of group play therapy: How to do it, how it works, whom it's best for* (pp. 86–104). San Francisco, CA: Jossey-Bass.

Betman, B. G. (2004). To see the world in a tray of sand: Using sandtray therapy with deaf children. *Odyssey, 5*(2), 16–20.

Bonds, M. S. (1995). Sandplay with inner-city Latino and African-American adolescents. (Doctoral dissertation, California School of Professional Psychology, Berkeley/Alameda). *Dissertation Abstract International*, AAT 9533887.

Boscolo, L., Cecchin, G., Hoffman, L., & Penn, P. (1987). *Milan systemic family therapy*. New York: Basic Books.

Bow, J. N. (1993). Overcoming resistance. In C. Schaefer (Ed.), *The therapeutic powers of play* (pp. 17–40). Northvale, NJ: Jason Aronson, Inc.

Bowen, M. (1976). Theory in the practice of psychotherapy. In P. Guerin (Ed.), *Family therapy: Theory and practice* (pp. 335–349). New York: Gardner Press.

Bowyer, L. R. (1970). *The Lowenfeld World Technique: Studies in personality*. New York: Pergamon Press.

Boyd-Franklin, N., Cleek, E., Wofsy, M., & Mundy, B. (2013). *Therapy in the real world: Effective treatments for challenging problems*. New York: Guilford Press.

Bradway, K., Signell, K. A., Spare, G. H., Stewart, C. T., Stewart, L. H., & Thompson, C. (1981). *Sandplay studies: Origins, theory, and practice*. San Francisco, CA: C.G. Jung Institute.

Bratton, S. (2015). The empirical support for play therapy: Strengths and limitations. In K. O'Connor, C. Schaefer, & L. Braverman (Eds.), *Handbook of play therapy* (2nd ed.), (pp. 651–668). New York: Wiley.

Brown, S., & Vaughan, C. (2009). *Play: How it shapes the brain, opens the imagination, and invigorates the soul*. New York: Avery Books.

Bühler, C. (1951a). The world test, a projective technique. *Journal of Child Psychiatry, 2*, 4–23.

Bühler, C. (1951b). The world test, a projective technique. *Journal of Child Psychiatry, 2*, 69–81.

Burke, V. (1996). Sandtray characteristics of schoolchildren by gender, ages seven through eleven. (Master thesis, Anchorage: University of Alaska Anchorage). *Dissertation Abstract International*, AAT 1380971.

Caesar, P. L., & Roberts, M. (1991). A conversational journey with clients and helpers: Therapist as tourist, not tour guide. *Journal of Strategic & Systemic Therapies, 10*(3–4), 38–51.

Caplan, F., & Caplan, T. (1974). *The power of play*. New York: Anchor Books.

Carnes-Holt, K., Meany-Walen, K., & Felton, A. (2014). Utilizing sandtray within the discrimination model of counselor supervision. *Journal of Creativity in Mental Health, 9*(4), 497–510.

Carrion, V., Wong, S., & Kletter, H. (2013). Update on neuroimaging and cognitive functioning in maltreatment-related pediatric PTSD: Treatment implications. *Journal of Family Violence, 28*(1), 53–61.

Chasin, R. (1989). Interviewing families with children: Guidelines and suggestions. *Journal of Psychotherapy and the Family, 5*(3/4), 15–30.

Cockle, S. (1993). Sandplay: A comparative study. *International Journal for Play Therapy, 2*(2), 1–17. doi: 10.1037/h0089349.

Cohen, J. (1988). *Statistical power analysis for the behavioral sciences* (2nd ed.). Hillside, NJ: Erlbaum.

Colapinto, J. (2000). Structural family therapy. In A. Horne (Ed.), *Family counseling and therapy* (3rd ed.), (pp. 140–169). Itasca, IL: Peacock.

Corey, M. S., Corey, G., & Corey, C. (2014). *Groups: Process and practice* (9th ed.). Belmont, CA: Brooks/Cole.

Dattilio, F. (2010). *Cognitive-behavioral therapy with couples and families: A comprehensive guide for clinicians*. New York: Guilford Press.

Dawson, L. S. (2011). Single-case analysis of sand tray therapy of depressive symptoms in early adolescence. Retrieved from ProQuest. (UMI Number: 3438887).

De Bellis, M., & Zisk, A. (2014). The biological effects of childhood trauma. *Child and Adolescent Psychiatric Clinics of North America, 23*(2), 185–222.

De Domenico, G. (1995). *Sandtray world play: A comprehensive guide to the use of the sandtray in psychotherapeutic and transformational settings*. Oakland, CA: Vision Quest Images.

De Domenico, G. (1999). Group sandtray-worldplay: New dimensions in sandplay therapy. In D. Sweeney & L. Homeyer (Eds.), *The handbook of group play therapy* (pp. 215–233). San Francisco, CA: Jossey-Bass.

de Shazer, S. (1988). *Clues: Investigating solutions in brief therapy*. New York: Norton & Company.

de Shazer, S., & Dolan, Y. (2007). *More than miracles: The state of the art of solution-focused brief therapy*. New York: Routledge.

Draper, K., Ritter, K., & Willingham, E. (2003). Sand tray group counseling with adolescents. *Journal for Specialists in Group Work, 28*(3), 244–260. doi: 10.1177/0193392203252030.

Duffy, S. (2015). Therapeutic stories and play in the sandtray for traumatized children: The moving stories method. In C. Malchiodi (Ed.), *Creative interventions with traumatized children* (2nd ed.), (pp. 150–168). New York: Guilford Press.

Eberts, S., & Homeyer, L. (2015). Processing sandtray from Gestalt and Adlerian perspectives. *International Journal of Play Therapy, 24*(3), 134–150. doi: 10.1037/a0039392.

Efstation, J. F., Patton, M. J., & Kardash, C. M. (1990). Measuring the working alliance in counselor supervision. *Journal of Counseling Psychology, 37*(3), 322–329.

Eichoff, L. (1952). Dreams in sand. *Journal of Mental Science, 98*, 235–243.

Ellis, A. (2008). Rational emotive behavior therapy. In R. Corsini & D. Wedding (Eds.), *Current psychotherapies* (8th ed.), (pp. 187–222). Belmont, CA: Thomson.

Fehr, S. (2017). *101 interventions in group therapy* (2nd ed.). New York: Routledge.

Fernando, C. (2006). Children of war in Sri Lanka: Promoting resilience through faith development. (Doctoral dissertation, University of Toronto (Canada), 2006). *Dissertation Abstract International*, AAT NR21881.

Fischer, K., & Bidell, T. (2006). Dynamic development of action, thought and emotion. In R. M. Lerner (Ed.), *Handbook of child psychology, Vol. 1: Theoretical models of human development* (6th ed.), (pp. 313–399). New York: Wiley.

Fishbane, M. (2013). *Loving with the brain in mind: Neurobiology and couple therapy*. New York: W.W. Norton & Company.

Flahive, M. W. (2005). Group sandtray therapy at school with preadolescents identified with behavioral difficulties. (Doctoral dissertation, Denton: University of North Texas, 2005). *Dissertation Abstract International*, AAT 3196148.

Flahive, M. W., & Ray, D. (2007). Effect of group sandtray therapy with preadolescents. *Journal for Specialists in Group Work, 32*(4), 362–382.

Freud, A. (1965). *The psycho-analytic treatment of children*. New York: International Universities Press.

Freud, S. (1909). *Analysis of a phobia in a five-year-old boy*. London: Hogarth Press.

Fujii, S. (1979). Retest reliability of the sand play techniques (1st report). *British Journal of Projective Psychology and Personality Study, 24*(2), 21–25.

Gaskill, R., & Perry, B. (2012). Child sexual abuse, traumatic experiences, and their impact on the developing brain. In P. Goodyear-Brown (Ed.), *Handbook of child sexual abuse: Identification, assessment and treatment* (pp. 29–48). Hoboken, NJ: John Wiley & Sons.

Gaskill, R., & Perry, B. (2014). The neurobiological power of play: Using the neurosequential model of therapeutics to guide play to guide play in the healing process. In C. Malchiodi & D. Crenshaw (Eds.), *Creative arts and play therapy for attachment problems* (pp. 178–196). New York: Guilford Press.

Gil, E. (1994). *Play in family therapy*. New York: Guilford.

Gil, E. (2003). Play genograms. In C. Sori & L. Heckler (Eds.), *The therapist's notebook for children and adolescents: Homework, handouts, and activities for use in psychotherapy* (pp. 49–56). New York: Haworth Press.

Gil, E. (2006). *Helping abused and traumatized children: Integrating directive and nondirective approaches*. New York: Guilford.

Gil, E. (2012). Trauma-focused integrated play therapy (TF-IPT). In P. Goodyear-Brown (Ed.), *Handbook of child sexual abuse: Identification, assessment, and treatment* (pp. 251–278). Hoboken, NJ: John Wiley & Sons.

Ginott, H. G. (1960). A rationale for selecting toys in play therapy. *Journal of Consulting Psychology, 24*(3), 243–246. doi: 10.1037/h0043980.

Glasse, C. (1995). *Teacher's guide: Sandplay in the classroom*. (no publisher listed) Del Diablo, Orinda, CA.

Gottman, J. M. (1994). *Why marriages succeed or fail*. New York: Simon and Schuster.

Grubbs, G. (1995). A comparative analysis of the sandplay process of sexually abused and nonclinical children. *The Arts in Psychotherapy, 22*(5), 429–446.

Guerin, P., Fay, L., Burden, S., & Kautto, J. (1987). *The evaluation and treatment of marital conflict*. New York: Basic Books.

Harper, J. (1991). Children's play: The differential effects of intrafamilial physical and sexual abuse. *Child Abuse & Neglect, 15*(1-2), 89–98.

Harter, S. (1985). *Manual for the self-perception profile for children*. Denver, CO: University of Denver.

Hendrix, H. (2010). *Doing imago relationship therapy: The definitive method*. New York: John Wiley & Sons.

Hick, S., & Bien, T. (Eds.) (2010). *Mindfulness and the therapeutic relationship*. New York: Guilford Press.

Homburger, E. (1938). Dramatic productions test. In H. Murray (Ed.), *Explorations in Personality* (pp. 554–582). New York: Oxford University Press.

Homeyer, L. (in press). Sandtray therapy: Use for all approaches. In B. Turner (Ed.), *International handbook of sandplay therapy*. East Sussex, UK: Routledge.

Homeyer, L., & Morrison, M. (2008). Play as therapy. *American Journal of Play, 1*(2), 210–228.

Homeyer, L., Poe, S., & DeFrance, E. (2004). *Group sandtray for at-risk children*. Unpublished manuscript.

Homeyer, L., & Sweeney, D. (1998). *Sandtray: A practical manual*. Royal Oak, MI: Self-Esteem Shop.

Homeyer, L., & Sweeney, D. (in press). Sandtray therapy: A variety of approaches. In B. Turner (Ed.), *The Routledge international handbook of sandplay therapy*. East Sussex, Great Britain: Routledge.

Howell, R. L. (1999). Children's concerns about danger and death: The influence of cognitive ability and bereavement. (Doctoral dissertation, California School of Professional Psychology, Berkeley/Alameda). *Dissertation Abstract International*, AAT 9907440.

Hug-Hellmuth, H. (1921). On the technique of child-analysis. *International Journal of Psychoanalysis, 2*, 287–305.

Hughes, S. C. (2004). The group sand tray: A case study. (Doctoral dissertation, Cincinnati: Union Institute and University). *Dissertation Abstract International*, AAT 3207605.

Jacobs, E., Schimmel, C., Masson, R., & Harvill, R. (2012). *Group counseling: Strategies and skills* (8th ed.). Belmont, CA: Brooks/Cole.

James, L., & Martin, D. (2002). Sand tray and group therapy: Helping parents cope. *The Journal of Specialist in Group Work, 27*(4), 390–405. doi: 10.180/714860201.

Johnson, S. M. (1996). *The practice of emotionally focused marital therapy: Creating connections*. New York, NY: Brunner/Mazel.

Johnson, S. M. (2004). *The practice of emotionally focused couple therapy: Creating connection* (2nd ed.). New York, NY: Brunner-Routledge.

Jones, L. E. (1986). *The development of structure in the world of expression: A cognitive-developmental analysis of children's "sand worlds."* Ann Arbor, MI: ProQuest UMI Dissertations.

Jung, C. G. (1928). *Contributions to analytical psychology.* New York, NY: Harcourt Brace.

Jung, C. G. (1971). *The portable Jung.* New York, NY: Viking Press.

Jung, C. G. (1977). *Symbols of transformation.* Princeton, NJ: Princeton University Press.

Kabat-Zinn, J. (1990). *Full catastrophe living: Using the wisdom of your body and mind to face stress, pain, and illness.* New York, NY: Bantam Books.

Kalff, D. (1971). *Sandplay: Mirror of a child's psyche.* San Francisco, CA: C.G. Jung Institute.

Kalff, D. (1980). *Sandplay: A psychotherapeutic approach to the psyche.* Santa Monica, CA: Sigo Press.

Kalff, D. (1981). Foreword. In K. Bradway, et al., (Eds.), *Sandplay studies: Origins, theory and practice.* San Francisco: C.G. Jung Institute.

Kalff, D. (2003). *Sandplay: A psychotherapeutic approach to the psyche.* Cloverdale, CA: Temenos Press.

Katz, A. (2010). Israeli Arab-Jewish sandtray group work: Creating a world together. *Psychotherapy and Politics International, 2*(8), 113–127. doi: 10.1002/ppi.

Keith, D., & Whitaker, C. (1981). Play therapy: A paradigm for work with families. *Journal of Marital and Family Therapy, 7*(3), 243–354.

Kestly, T. (2001). Group sandplay in elementary schools. In A. Drews, L. Carey, & C. Schaefer (Eds.), *School-based play therapy* (pp. 329–349). New York, NY: Wiley.

Kestly, T. (2010). Group sandplay in elementary schools. In A. Drews, L. Carey, & C. Schaefer (Eds.), *School-based play therapy* (pp. 257–281). Hoboken, NJ: John Wiley & Sons.

Kestly, T. (2014). *The interpersonal neurobiology of play: Brain-building interventions for emotional well-being.* New York, NY: W.W. Norton & Company.

Kestly, T. (2015). Sandtray and storytelling in play therapy. In D. Crenshaw & A. Stewart (Eds.), *Play therapy: A comprehensive guide to theory and practice* (pp. 156–170). New York, NY: Guilford Press.

Klein, M. (1932). *The psycho-analysis of children.* London: Hogarth Press.

Korner, S., & Brown, G. (1990). Exclusion of children from family psychotherapy: Family therapists' beliefs and practices. *Journal of Family Psychology, 3*(4), 420–430.

Kottman, T. (1999). Group applications of Adlerian play therapy. In D. Sweeney & L. Homeyer (Eds.), *The handbook of group play therapy: How to do it, how it works, whom it's best for* (pp. 65–85). San Francisco, CA: Jossey-Bass.

Kramer, E. (1972). *Art as therapy with children.* New York, NY: Schocken Books.

Kwiatkowska, H. (1978). *Family therapy and evaluation through art.* Springfield, IL: Charles C. Thomas Publisher.

Lacroix, L., Rousseau, C., Gauthier, M., Singh, A., Giguère, N., & Lemzoudi, Y. (2007). Immigrant and refugee preschoolers' sandplay representations of the tsunami. *The Arts in Psychotherapy, 34*(2), 99–113.

Landreth, G. (2012). *Play therapy: The art of the relationship* (3rd ed.). New York, NY: Routledge.

Landreth, G., & Sweeney, D. (1999). The freedom to be: Child-centered group play therapy. In D. Sweeney & L. Homeyer (Eds.), *The handbook of group play therapy: How to do it, how it works, whom it's best for* (pp. 39–64). San Francisco: Jossey-Bass, Inc. Publishers.

Lanius, R., Williamson, P., Densmore, M., Boksman, K., Neufeld, R., Gati, J., & Menon, R. (2004). The nature of traumatic memories: A 4-T fMRI functional connectivity analysis. *Archives of General Psychiatry, 161*(1), 36–44.

Linehan, M. (1993). *Skills training manual for treating borderline personality disorder.* New York, NY: Guilford Press.

Linehan, M. (2015a). *DBT skills training manual* (2nd ed.). New York, NY: Guilford Press.

Linehan, M. (2015b). *DBT skills training handouts and worksheets* (2nd ed.). New York, NY: Guilford Press.

Linehan, M., & Wilks, C. (2015). The course and evolution of dialectical behavior therapy. *American Journal of Psychotherapy, 69*(2), 97–110.

Lowenfeld, M., & Dukes, E. (1938). Play therapy and child guidance: Correspondence section. *The British Medical Journal*, Dec. 17, 2, 1281.

Lowenfeld, M. (1939). The world pictures of children: A method of recording and studying them. *British Journal of Medical Psychology, 18*(1), 65–101.

Lowenfeld, M. (1950). The nature and use of the Lowenfeld World Technique in work with children and adults. *The Journal of Psychology, 30*(2), 325–331.

Lowenfeld, M. (1967). On normal emotional and intellectual development of children. Lecture presented at St. Edmund's College, Ware, England.

Lowenfeld, M. (1979a). *Understanding children's sandplay: Lowenfeld's world technique.* London: George Allen & Urwin.

Lowenfeld, M. (1979b). *The world technique.* London: Allen & Unwin.

Lowenfeld, M. (1993). *Understanding children's sandplay: The world technique.* Great Britain: Antony Rowe Ltd. (Originally published as *The World Technique*, Chippenham: George Allen & Unwin, 1979).

Lu, L., Peterson, F., Lacroix, L., & Rousseau, C. (2010). Stimulating creative play in children with autism through sandplay. *The Arts in Psychotherapy, 37*(1), 55–64.

Lumry, G. K. (1951). Study of world test characteristics as a basis for discrimination between various clinical categories. *Journal of Child Psychiatry, 2*(1), 24–35.

Madanes, C. (1984). *Behind the one-way mirror: Advances in the practice of strategic therapy.* San Francisco, CA: Jossey-Bass.

Malchiodi, C. (2015). *Creative interventions with traumatized children* (2nd ed.). New York, NY: Guilford Press.

Markos, P., Coker, J. K., & Jones, W. P. (2008). Play in supervision. *Journal of Creativity in Mental Health, 2*(3), 3–15. doi: 10.1300/J456v02n03_02.

Mason, L. B. (1986). Assessing couple integration with the sandplay method (marriage). (Doctoral dissertation, University of California, Berkeley). *Dissertation Abstract International*, AAT 8624858.

McCarthy, D. (2006). Sandplay therapy and the body in trauma recovery. In L. Carey (Ed.), *Expressive and creative arts methods for trauma survivors* (pp. 165–180). London: Jessica Kingsley Publishers.

McCown, S. (2008). An inclusive sandtray friendship group in an elementary setting: A descriptive study. (Doctoral dissertation, Minneapolis: Capella University). Available from ProQuest Dissertations and Theses database (UMI No. 3304142).

McGoldrick, M., Gerson, R., & Petty, S. (2008). *Genograms: Assessment and intervention* (3rd ed.). New York, NY: W.W. Norton & Company.

Miller, C., & Boe, J. (1990). Tears into diamonds: Transformation of child psychic trauma through sandplay and storytelling. *The Arts in Psychotherapy, 17*(3), 247–257.

Miller, W., & Rollnick, S. (2002). *Motivational interviewing: Preparing people for change* (2nd ed.). New York, NY: Guilford Press.

Miller, W., & Rollnick, S. (2013). *Motivational interviewing: Preparing people for change* (3rd ed.). New York: Guilford Press.

Millikin, J., & Johnson, S. (2000). Telling tales: Disquisition in emotionally focused therapy. *Journal of Family Psychotherapy, 11*(1), 75–79.

Mills, J., & Crowley, R. (1986). *Therapeutic metaphors for children and the child within.* New York, NY: Brunner/Mazel.

Minuchin, S. (1974). *Families and family therapy.* Cambridge, MA: Harvard University Press.

Mitchell, R. R., & Friedman, H. S. (1994). *Sandplay: Past, present and future.* New York, NY: Routledge.

Monakes, S., Garza, Y., Weisner, V., & Watts, R. (2011). Implementing Adlerian sandtray therapy with adult male substance abuse offenders: A phenomenology inquiry. *Journal of Addictions & Offender Counseling, 31*(2), 94–107.

Monson, C., & Shnaider, P. (2014). Trauma-focused interventions: Cognitive techniques and treatment packages. In C. Monson & P. Shnaider (Eds.), *Treating PTSD with cognitive-behavioral therapies: Interventions that work* (pp. 51–79). Washington, DC: American Psychological Association.

Moon, B. (2015). *Ethical issues in art therapy* (3rd ed.). Springfield, IL: Charles C. Thomas Publisher.

Nasab, H. M., & Alipor, Z. M. (2015). The effectiveness of sandplay therapy in reducing symptoms of separation anxiety in children 5 to 7 years old. *Journal UMP Social Sciences and Technology Management, 3*(2), 5–10.

Neill, T. (2006). *Helping others help children: Clinical supervision of child psychotherapy.* Washington, DC: American Psychological Association.

Nelson, K. Z. (2011). The sandtray technique for Swedish children 1945–1960: Diagnostics, psychotherapy and processes of individuation. *Paedagogical Historica, 47*(6), 825–840. doi: 10.1080/00309230.2011.621204.

Nichols, M. (2013). *Family therapy: Concepts and methods* (10th Ed.). Boston: Pearson.

Nims, D. (2007). Integrating play therapy techniques into solution-focused brief therapy. *International Journal of Play Therapy, 16*(1), 54–68.

No, S., & Kim, N. (2013). The effects of sandplay therapy on anxiety, interpersonal stress, and salivary cortisol levels of university students with ADHD tendencies. *Journal of Symbols & Sandplay Therapy, 4*(1), 9–15. doi: 10.12964/jsst.13002.

Oaklander, V. (1999). Group play therapy from a Gestalt therapy perspective. In D. Sweeney & L. Homeyer (Eds.), *The handbook of group play therapy: How to do it, how it works, whom it's best for* (pp. 162–175). San Francisco, CA: Jossey-Bass.

Paone, T., Malott, J., Gao, J., & Kinda, G. (2015). Using sandplay to address students' reactions to multicultural counselor training. *International Journal of Play Therapy, 24*(4), 190–204. doi: 10.1037/a0039813.

Papp, P., Silverstein, O., & Carter, E. (1973). Family sculpting in preventive work with well families. *Family Process, 12*(2), 197–212.

Parker, N., & O'Brien, P. (2011). Play therapy-reaching the child with autism. *International Journal of Special Education, 26*(1), 80–87.

Perls, F. (1969). *Gestalt therapy verbatim.* Moab, UT: Real People Press.

Perry, B. (2006). Applying principles of neurodevelopment to clinical work with maltreated and traumatized children: The neurosequential model therapeutics. In N. B. Webb (Ed.), *Working with Traumatized youth in child welfare* (pp. 27–52). New York, NY: Guilford Press.

Perry, B. (2009). Examining child maltreatment through a neurodevelopmental lens: Clinical applications of the neurosequential model of therapeutics. *Journal of Loss and Trauma, 14*(4), 240–255.

Perry, B., & Pate, J. (1994). Neurodevelopment and the psychobiological roots of post-traumatic stress disorder. In L. Koziol & C. Stout (Eds.), *The neuropsychology of mental disorders: A practical guide* (pp. 129–146). Springfield, IL: Charles C. Thomas Publisher.

Petruk, L. (1996). Creating a world in the sand: A pilot study of normative data for employing the sand tray as a diagnostic tool with children. (Master's thesis, Southwest Texas State University, San Marcos, Texas).

Plotkin, L. (2011). Children's adjustment following parental divorce: How effective is sandtray play therapy? (Doctoral dissertation, Minneapolis: Capella University). Retrieved from ProQuest. (UMI Number: 3466536).

Raftopoulos, M. (2015). The use of jewels in the sandplay therapy of children with and without abuse histories. *Journal of Sandplay Therapy, 24*(1), 47–68.

Ray, D. (2006). Evidenced-based play therapy. In C. Schaefer & H. Kaduson (Eds.), *Contemporary play therapy: Theory, research and practice* (pp. 136–157). New York, NY: Guilford Press.

Ray, D. (2015). Research in play therapy: Empirical support for practice. In D. Crenshaw & A. Stewart (Eds.), *Play therapy: A comprehensive guide to theory and practice* (pp. 467–482). New York, NY: Guilford Press.

Reynolds, C. R., & Kamphaus, R. W. (1992). *Behavior assessment system for children: Manual.* Circle Pines, MN: American Guidance.

Rothbaum, B., & Foa, E. (1996). Cognitive-behavioral therapy for posttraumatic stress disorder. In B. van der Kolk, A. McFarlane, & L. Weisaeth (Eds.), *Traumatic stress* (pp. 491–509). New York, NY: Guilford Press.

Roubenzadeh, S., Abendin, A., & Heidari, M. (2012). Effectiveness of sand tray short term group therapy with grieving youth. *Procedia: Social and Behavioral Sciences, 69*, 2131–2136. doi: 10.1016/j.sbspro.2012.12.177.

Rousseau, C., Benoit, M., Lacroix, L., & Gauthier, M. (2009). Evaluation of a sandplay program for preschoolers in a multiethnic neighborhood. *Journal of Child Psychology and Psychiatry, 50*(6), 743–750. doi: 10.1111/j.1469–7610.2008.02003.x.

Ryce-Menuhin, J. (1992). *Jungian sandplay: The wonderful therapy.* New York, NY: Routledge.

Schaefer, C. (1994). Play therapy for psychic trauma in children. In K. O'Connor & C. Schaefer (Eds.), *Handbook of play therapy,* Volume 2 (pp. 297–318). New York, NY: John Wiley & Sons.

Schore, D. J. (2009). Right-brain affect regulation: An essential mechanism of development, trauma, dissociation, and psychotherapy. In D. Fosha, M. Solomon, & D. Siegel (Eds.), *The healing power of emotion: Integrating relationships, body and mind: A dialogue among scientists and clinicians* (pp. 112–144). New York, NY: Norton & Company.

Shen, Y. (2006). The impact of school-based group sandtray counseling on the self-esteem of young adolescent girls. (Doctoral dissertation, Commerce: Texas A&M University). *Dissertation Abstracts International,* AAT 3245238.

Shen, Y., & Armstrong, S. A. (2008). Impact of group sandtray therapy on the self-esteem of young adolescent girls. *Journal for Specialists in Group Work, 33*(2), 118–137.

Siegel, D. J. (1999). *The developing mind: How relationship and the brain interact to shape who we are.* New York, NY: Guilford Press.

Siegel, D. J. (2003). An interpersonal neurobiology of psychotherapy: The developing mind and the resolution of trauma. In M. Solomon & D. Siegel (Eds.), *Healing trauma: Attachment, mind, body, and brain* (pp. 1–56). New York, NY: W.W. Norton & Company.

Siegelman, E. (1990). *Metaphor and meaning in psychotherapy.* New York, NY: The Guilford Press.

Siever, R. (1988). *Sand.* New York, NY: W. H. Freeman & Company.

Sjolund, M., & Schaefer, C. (1994). The Erica method of sand play diagnosis and assessment. In K. J. O'Connor & C. E. Schaefer (Eds.), *Handbook of play therapy: Advances and innovations,* Volume 2 (pp. 231–252). New York, NY: Wiley.

Sonstegard, M. (1998). The theory and practice of Adlerian group counseling and psychotherapy. *The Journal of Individual Psychology, 54*(2), 217–250.

Spare, G. (1981). Are there any rules (musings of a peripatetic sandplayer). In K. Bradway, K. Signell, G. Spare, C. Stewart, L. Steward, & C. Thompson (Eds.), *Sandplay studies: Origins, theory and practice* (pp. 195–208). San Francisco: C.G. Jung Institute.

Stahl, B., & Goldstein, E. (2010). *A mindfulness-based stress reduction workbook.* Oakland, CA: New Harbinger Publications.

Stark, M., Garza, Y., Bruhn, R., & Ane, P. (2015). Student perception of sandtray in solution-focused supervision. *Journal of Creativity and Mental Health, 10*(1), 2–17. doi: 10.1080/15401383.2014.917063.

Steinhardt, L. (1997). Beyond blue: The implications of blue as the color of the inner surface of the sandtray in sandplay. *The Arts in Psychotherapy, 24*(5), 455–469.

Swank, J., & Lenes, E. (2013). An exploratory inquiry of sandtray group experiences with adolescent females in an alternative school. *Journal for Specialists in Group Work, 38*(4), 330–348. doi: 10.1080/09133922.2013.835013.

Sweeney, D. (1997). *Counseling children through the world of play.* Wheaton, IL: Tyndale House Publishers.

Sweeney, D. (1999). Introduction. In L. Carey (Ed.), *Sandplay with children and families* (pp. ix–xxvi). Northvale, NJ: Jason Aronson, Inc.

Sweeney, D. (2002). Sandplay with couples. In R. Watts (Ed.), *Techniques in marriage and family counseling,* Volume 2 (pp. 95–104). Alexandria, VA: American Counseling Association.

Sweeney, D. (2011). Group play therapy. In C. E. Schaefer (Ed.), *Foundations of play therapy* (2nd ed.), (pp. 227–252). New York, NY: Wiley.

Sweeney, D., Baggerly, J., & Ray, D. (2014). *Group play therapy: A dynamic approach.* New York: Routledge Publishers.

Sweeney, D., & Homeyer, L. (Eds.) (1999). *Handbook of group play therapy.* San Francisco: Jossey-Bass, Inc. Publishers.

Sweeney, D., Minnix, G., & Homeyer, L. (2003). Using the sandtray for lifestyle analysis. *Journal of Individual Psychology, 59*(4), 376–387.

Sweeney, D., & Rocha, S. (2000). Using play therapy to assess family dynamics. In R. Watts (Ed.), *Techniques in marriage and family counseling,* Volume 1 (pp. 33–47). Alexandria, VA: American Counseling Association.

Taylor, E. R. (2009). Sandtray and solution-focused therapy. *International Journal of Play Therapy, 18*(1), 56–68.

Teicher, M., Tomoda, A., & Andersen, S. (2006). Neurobiological consequences of early tress and childhood maltreatment. In R. Yehuda (Ed.), *Psychobiology of posttraumatic stress disorder: A decade of progress* (pp. 313–323). Boston, MA: Blackwell Publishing.

Thompson, C. (1990). Variations on a theme by Lowenfeld: Sandplay in focus. In K. Bradway (Ed.), *Sandplay studies: Origins, theory and practice* (pp. 5–20). San Francisco, CA: C.G. Jung Institute.

Thompson, C. L., & Rudolph, L. B. (2000). *Counseling children.* Belmont, CA: Wadsworth/Thomson Learning.

van der Kolk, B. (2002). Assessment and treatment of complex PTSD. In R. Yehuda (Ed.), *Treating trauma survivors with PTSD* (pp. 127–156). Washington, DC: American Psychiatric Publishing.

van der Kolk, B. (2006). Clinical implications of neuroscience research in PTSD. In R. Yehuda (Ed.), *Psychobiology of posttraumatic stress disorder: A decade of progress* (pp. 277–293). Boston: Blackwell Publishing.

van der Kolk, B. (2014). *The body keeps the score: Brain, mind, and body in the healing of trauma.* New York, NY: Penguin Group.

Viers, D. (2007). *The group therapist's notebook: Homework, handouts, and activities for use in psychotherapy.* New York, NY: Routledge.

Weeks, G., & L'Abate, L. (1982). *Paradoxical psychotherapy: Theory and practice with individuals, couples, and families.* New York, NY: Brunner/Mazel.

Weinrib, E. (1983). *Images of self: The sandplay therapy process.* Boston, MA: Sigo Press.

Wells, H. G. (1911). *Floor games.* New York, NY: Arno Press. (Originally published in England. First U.S. edition, 1912, Boston, MA).

Wen, Z., Risheng, Z., Haslam, D., & Zhiling, J. (2011). The effects of restricted group sandplay on interpersonal issues of college students in China. *The Arts in Psychotherapy, 38*(4), 281–289. doi: 10.1016/j.aip.2011.08.008.

Wheat, R. (1995). Help children work through emotional difficulties—sandtrays are great! *Young Children, 51*(1), 82–83.

White, M. (2007). *Maps of narrative practice.* New York, NY: W.W. Norton & Company.

Wylie, M. (2004). The limits of talk: Bessel van der Kolk wants to transform the treatment of trauma. *Psychotherapy Networker, 28*, 30–41.

Yalom, I. (2005). *The theory and practice of group psychotherapy* (5th ed.). New York, NY: Basic Books.

Zarzaur, M. (2004). The effectiveness of sandtray therapy versus classroom behavior management on the improvement of school behavior of kindergarten through fourth-grade students. (Master's thesis, Memphis: The University of Memphis). *Dissertation Abstract International,* AAT 3153961.

Index

Note: Page numbers in italics indicate figures.

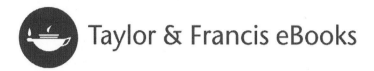
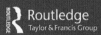